PRAISE
TRY NEW

MW01015229

"Parents who are frustrated about their child's eating, who feel at a loss about what to do, and who are worried their child isn't eating the "right" foods will find relief in this book. Jill not only walks parents through the process of helping their child taste and discover new foods, but she also arms them with the knowledge and encouragement they truly need to be better feeders. This is an outstanding resource!"

— Sally Kuzemchak, MS, RD, author of *The 101 Healthiest Foods For Kids* and founder of RealMomNutrition.com

"The beauty of Jill Castle's workbook edition of *Try New Food* is that it feels as though Jill is sitting with you at the family table. Picky eating doesn't just impact the child, it changes the whole family dynamic. Jill's strategies address the big picture by supporting parents in the process of helping kids taste and learn to love a variety of foods. Yes, your child will become more adventurous, but just as important, the process will bring joy back to your family table once again."

— Melanie Potock, MA, CCC-SLP, pediatric feeding specialist and author of *Adventures in Veggieland: Help Your Kids Learn to Love Vegetables with 100 Easy Activities and Recipes*

"All parents want their children to willingly try new food but some kids need more support. Try New Food provides the steps, framework, and strategy parents need to help their children get there. It's a must read for any parent of a cautious eater!"

— Maryann Jacobsen, MS, RD, author of *From Picky to Powerful*

"This is the book I wish I'd had when I started on my own journey as a parent. Written by one of the country's foremost authorities on feeding kids (who is a mother of four herself), *Try New Food* is packed with practical advice, doable tips, and a user-friendly workbook. Perhaps best of all, the stories and anecdotes will make you feel like you aren't the only one with a picky kid and assure you that it won't be like this forever."

— Katie Sullivan Morford, MS, RD, author of *Rise & Shine* and *Best Lunch Box Ever*

"*Try New Food: How to Help Picky Eaters Taste, Eat & Like New Foods* is the essential workbook for parents who want their children to have a positive relationship with a wide range of food. This book is packed with tools and practical strategies to reduce mealtime stress and picky eating tendencies. Parents learn simple tips to introduce new food to their child with confidence and fun! As a Registered Dietitian and mother of two children, I find this workbook to be very helpful with my own family. It is a must-have resource for every parent as well as any health care professional who works with children."

— Clancy Harrison, TEDx Speaker, Food Justice Advocate, Registered Dietitian

"Jill hits the mark with the workbook edition of Try New Food! It is a practical, accurate and timely resource for both parents and professionals. The workbook actively engages the reader with sound feeding advice along with space devoted for reflections to promote a positive feeding relationship. As a pediatric dietitian, I am thrilled to have this resource to recommend to families!"

— Karen McGrail, MEd, RDN, Director of the John Stalker Institute of Food and Nutrition

"Jill Castle's *Try New Food Workbook* is the exact resource parents need to take the stress out of family mealtimes. She demystifies what picky eating really is and helps parents take responsibility for their role in their children's eating (or lack thereof). I particularly love her practical, eye-opening exercises and her actionable tips for ensuring children get the balance they need in their diets while making mealtimes something everyone in the family can look forward to. I highly recommend the workbook for parents who want to bring more calm into their feeding style and model healthy behaviors with food for their children."

— Alexia Vernon, Keynote Speaker, Author, Speaking Coach & Trainer

TRY NEW FOOD

HOW TO HELP PICKY EATERS TASTE, EAT & LIKE NEW FOODS

The Workbook Edition

BY JILL CASTLE, MS, RDN

Editing by Arnetta Jackson
Cover and book design by Streetlight Graphics

Published in the United States by Nourished Child Press
www.JillCastle.com

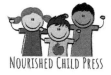

NOURISHED CHILD PRESS

To Grace, Madeline, Caroline and Ben,

I'm forever grateful for the opportunity to nourish and nurture you. You've taught me more than you will ever know.

Love, Mom

TABLE OF CONTENTS

PROLOGUE

A FEW YEARS AGO, I DECIDED to create a resource that would highlight and showcase the way I work with kids in my practice who are unwilling to try new food. I wrote *Try New Food: Help New Eaters, Picky Eaters and Extreme Picky Eaters Taste, Eat and Like New Foods*. You can imagine after 25+ years of working with families, I've seen a lot, and figured out some strategies that are positive and productive in this area of parenting and feeding—strategies that honor Ellyn Satter's Division of Responsibility with Feeding, while also preserving and giving attention to food, nutrients, and your child's personality.

Try New Food has been a welcome resource for many of you. It has helped you with practical steps, new foods to offer your child, and perhaps even given you the opportunity to pause and reflect on your role in your child's eating. You've told me it's given you fresh ideas; it's calmed you down; it's given you goals and a pathway to gently forge a plan.

However, since the book released, I wanted to make it even more useful and helpful. So that's what I've done. I've added reflections and exercises, so that you can take time to sort out your child's reactions, his or her food preferences, how things are progressing (or not), and your own feelings about feeding your child. I provide you more background on the *why* behind fussy eating; an opportunity to look at your child's experience with food, and embellish the steps and strategies to help your child try new food. In essence, I've created a workbook to transform the way you think about your child, the way you interact and handle food with your child, and help you "work through" the tricky, joy-robbing experience of raising a child who won't try new food.

Try New Food: How to Help Picky Eaters Taste, Eat & Like New Foods is my attempt to walk with you as you embark on this journey. I hope it transforms your thoughts, ideas, and actions!

~Jill

INTRODUCTION

WHEN I HAD MY FIRST daughter, I naively thought she would be a food-loving experimentalist, excited to try all kinds of new and exotic food. She was never that until she was much older.

In fact, she was "my little birdie." She sat in her high chair and picked a bit of this and a bit of that to eat, then said she was "all done" and wanted to get down. My biggest mistake was allowing her to toddle around with a sippy cup of whole milk all day. Whole milk was my crutch—and hers. She didn't eat much at meals, so I made sure she had access to milk whenever she wanted it. Why was this a mistake, you wonder? By twelve months, she was barely meeting her expected weight gain, and by eighteen months, she was anemic.

Picky eating and its complications can catch *any* parent by surprise, creeping up over time, and stealing the joy from feeding your child. Helping your child try new food is one parenting obligation you need to fulfill to successfully raise a healthy eater. While this book is devoted to helping you help your child try new food, you need to know all the elements of success, including a good understanding of picky eating.

BEHIND DOOR #3: THE OPTION YOU NEED TO KNOW

If you have high expectations for your child's adventurous spirit around food (like I did), you may find yourself feeling terribly disappointed. Picky eaters can be frustrating and worrisome. While you have a heart for your child's struggle with food, it can be very inconvenient and annoying. Let's be real. Children who shy away from trying a new food stir up some stressful emotions. These feelings—guilt, shame, frustration, fear, anxiety, and embarrassment—show up in your day-to-day reality. And they can negatively affect your feeding interactions.

When you seek help for picky eating, you'll hear two primary pieces of advice. One common response is to wait until your child grows out of it. Most parents I meet have heard this advice and they're over it. The second piece of advice is to take action, and well, somehow *make* your child eat. You've probably heard your fair share of *Try this food, it worked for my little guy* or *Did you try blending vegetables into xyz food?*

You need to know there is a third, better piece of advice. One that encourages you to be a positive, tuned in parent so that your child not only tries new food, but also develops healthy eating habits for life.

WHAT IS PICKY EATING?

The definition of picky eating runs the gamut. When I look at the scientific research, there are many variations on the term picky eating, as well as how it is defined. Because of the variability in how picky eating is defined, the prevalence rates and outcomes associated with picky eating aren't streamlined. In other words, they are all over the map.

For the purpose of this workbook, I'm using the definition outlined by a 2015 review article in *Appetite*.[1]

Picky eating (also known as fussy, faddy, finicky, or choosy eating) is characterized by an unwillingness to eat familiar foods or to try new foods, as well as strong food preferences severe enough to interfere with daily routines to an extent that is problematic to the parent, child, or parent–child relationship.

Picky eating can look wildly different from child to child. For example:

- One child may want hot dogs for three or four days in a row, while another may eat them for months on end.

- One child may grimace when he tastes broccoli, while another may gag and vomit.

- Some children will branch out and eventually try a new food, especially when there aren't other options, while another child refuses to eat, preferring to go to bed hungry.

- One child will eat at school, but when offered the same foods at home, will turn up his nose.

Picky eating commonly reveals itself between ages two and six. Somewhere during that time, children may refuse new foods, get stuck on their favorite foods, and even be fearful of foods they don't recognize. This typically translates to eating less food, having quite a bit of repetition in the diet, and the onset of mealtime battles.

On the topic of picky eating, you'll find some fancy terminology thrown around to describe features of pickiness. I want you to know what these terms mean:

Food neophobia: A reluctance to eat and/or fear of new food

Food jag: Repeatedly requesting and eating the same foods

Early satiety: A feeling of fullness early in the meal which triggers a child to stop eating

Picky eating seems to affect girls and boys equally.[1] The presence of siblings and older moms have been shown to be protective against the development of picky eating.[1] Most studies show that food intake is reduced during the picky eating phase, and diet quality (nutritional content) suffers for many children.[1] Specifically, there is lower fruit and vegetable intake, lower vitamin and mineral intake, and fewer whole grains and fiber consumption.[1] These factors put children who are picky eaters at higher risk for being underweight and having poor growth, or for being overweight.[1]

In the United States, picky eating reportedly occurs in 10%-50% of children, depending on the age of the child and the study. One study found that 50% of two-year-olds were picky, while three- and four-year-olds showed a prevalence of 21 percent.[2,3] Almost 11% of nine-year-old children were found to be picky eaters.[4]

Picky eating tends to resolve itself over time. Eventually, children try new food and even add back those rejected, but previously liked, foods. Yet, not every reformed picky eater turns into a healthy eater. Those early food preferences and eating habits can get in the way of healthy eating. You need to know the key ingredients that make it more likely you'll raise a healthy eater for life. This workbook will help you do just that. Your child can become more adventurous and less fearful of new foods. That's good news!

However, for some kids, picky eating will be long and drawn out. But while it may have a stronghold for years, it will get better. For others, picky eating won't seem to ever resolve, and will look like it's getting worse with time. For them, the fear of trying new food and eating a bland, limited diet will be their reality unless more help is received.

MY CHILD WON'T TRY NEW FOOD

Samantha couldn't get her child to try anything new. She tried everything—sneaking spinach into smoothies, bribing with dessert, even punishing her child. "No matter what I do, Alex just won't even try. He looks at the food and either complains or completely ignores it," said Samantha. "I know if he would just try it, he'd like it!"

I hear this all the time—frustration with the child who simply zips those lips and won't even make a move to try new food. It's frustrating! You know if your child would just have a taste, she'd probably like it. Just a tiny bite. Even a little lick. If she could just do that, chances are she would break through this cycle of eating the same foods, over and over. Chances are, she'd overcome her unwillingness to try new food. Chances are, she'd *change*.

I know this self-talk all too well. I did it myself! It goes something like this:

If I could just get my child to try new food, she would like it.

She can't be meeting her nutritional needs…she eats nothing healthy!

I wish she would become more adventurous (like her friend, my niece, the kids in her class…)

If she would be more open, our family meals would be more pleasant rather than full of meltdowns and drama.

If she would try new food, I wouldn't have to make her something else to eat every night.

To add insult to injury, you know she likes a particular food, but she won't touch the slight variation of it, even though her liked food is part of the ingredient list. For example, your child likes strawberry jam but she won't touch fresh strawberries or any other food made with them. It's downright mind boggling.

Yet, you keep trying. And that's a good thing. But sometimes, 'trying' can get us, and our kids, into trouble.

WHY IT'S SO CHALLENGING TO INTRODUCE NEW FOOD

One of the jobs of being a parent or caretaker is to expose your child to a variety of different foods. This broadens your child's palate, offers more nutrition, and helps him like a lot of different foods in the future. My guess is you've probably heard the variety message, over and over.

Yet, if you're following the advice to wait until your child outgrows picky eating, then you're probably not too concerned with introducing food variety. In fact, you're likely in what I call "hoping and praying" mode, waiting for some magical experience to transform your child into a broccoli-requesting fiend. Or, if you're in the take action camp, you're probably bombarding your child with comments, questions, and bribes to take a bite of broccoli. I'm here to show you there's a much better way. One that ditches that old, ineffective advice and helps you raise a healthy eater while nurturing and nourishing your child, inside and out.

We can all acknowledge the challenges involved in introducing new foods to a child. Part of the difficulty is that their development may be complicating things. Toddlers want to separate and be independent of their parent. "No," and "I do it" are common phrases of this age. This goes for everything, food and eating included. In fact, exerting independence with food is one of the primary ways they establish their autonomy (along with potty-training).

I had this experience with my own daughter. She got stuck on raisins, pancakes, and milk. Those were her favorite foods (in addition to hot dogs). She asked for them all the time, and would occasionally throw a fit if she couldn't have them. The only time she was open to try something new was when she sat on my husband's lap and picked around at his meal. She tried salmon, steak, and baked potato. Because she had moved away from her own meal, there was no pressure to eat something on my husband's plate, so she could explore, touch, and taste on her own terms.

When you think about the toddler, the child, and even the adolescent, getting them to do anything you want them to do is, in part, successful when it's their idea. In other words, motivation is greater when they are part of the decision-making, or it's on their terms. Somehow, when we are in the thick of feeding our kids, we can lose sight of this fact.

WHY IS EVERY CHILD I KNOW ADVENTUROUS?

While this may seem the case, few children are considered "adventurous," or willing to accept *any* food offered to them. A small percentage of kids are timid and shy with food. Most kids fall somewhere in between and learn to taste, eat, and like new food over time.

It's no surprise that an unwillingness to try new food is exactly what gets frustrating for parents. Kids need a familiarization period. This takes time, consistency, and persistence. Not only that, it's riddled with food acceptance and food refusal. If your expectations are higher than what your child can meet, you may struggle with disappointment. You may even delve into old habits like hiding vegetables in food like spaghetti sauce. While this isn't terrible, it can facilitate distrust.

If you have a child who is moving through the usual stages of picky eating, a child who seems to take longer to warm up to new foods, or a child who gets stuck eating from a short list of foods, then *how* you introduce new foods is critical. Why? Because *how* you feed can help or hinder the picky eater, and can slow down or speed up the process of moving through it.

Don't worry, that's what this book is all about. I want to make sure you know the ins and outs of introducing and adding new foods to your child's diet, no matter his personality, temperament, or eating challenges. I'll be covering this and more as we work through this book.

THE PERFECT STORM FOR PICKY EATING

Two aspects about kids will always throw a wrench into the process of introducing new foods: their temperament and their developmental stage. We rarely talk about these, but I believe you have to know *how* to work *with* your child in order to move him along the path to trying new food.

Here's what I mean: If you have a stubborn, dig-in-my-heels kind of kid, he'll probably fight you every step of the way. A child with this temperament needs to be in charge. That's not to say he *really* needs to be in charge (and he shouldn't be), but he needs to *feel* he is. A child with an opposite temperament, one who is more compliant and wants to please his parents, will be more likely to do what is asked of him, perhaps appearing to be adventurous, or a good eater.

The other piece is an even bigger player. The developmental stage is predictable and progressive. This is both good and bad news. It's predictable; which means that picky eating will probably happen between the ages of 2 and 6 years, just like the science says it will. The intensity and degree of pickiness will of course vary from child to child, but the likelihood it will happen is strong (that's the bad news). The good news is that development is progressive. You will both eventually get through it.

WHY I WROTE THIS BOOK

I wrote *Try New Food*: *How to Help Picky Eaters Taste, Eat & Like New Foods* because the topic of *how* to get kids to try new food is one of the most frequent questions I get from parents as a pediatric nutrition expert. Parents tell me how stressed they are about their child's unwillingness to taste food. They tell me that picky eating is taking over the dinner table. Picky eating is stealing the joy from being together, eating a meal, and being a parent.

I've been working with picky eaters in my private practice for years. Over decades, the complexity of picky eating has changed. In past years, picky eating mainly centered around children not eating their vegetables. Fast forward: other foods like protein sources, dairy foods, and fruit became equally concerning for parents. Before, it was about bitter and spicy flavors, and foods not touching each other. Today, it's about texture, smell, super-tasters, and sensory-integration.

Simultaneously, I found I was talking less about food as the solution to pickiness. I was spending more time on the feeding interaction between parent and child as a primary factor in helping families live with picky eating—and overcome it—without further complicating the situation.

I was also seeing incredibly complex picky eaters in my practice: Older children that ate only 20 or 30 foods; kids who were underweight; ones who had serious nutrient deficiencies; and others who were experiencing tremendous anxiety around food and eating. In an attempt to help, I developed an approach to reduce negative feeding interactions, while helping parents ease their child into tasting and eventually eating new foods. I call it The Nourished Path™ to New Foods.

I wrote this workbook to help you help your child try new food. I crafted this to help you use the most positive feeding strategies so you can avoid unnecessarily prolonging your child's picky eating, or making it worse. And I wrote it to help you recognize the more complex picky eater, so your child can get the individualized attention and intervention she needs, if warranted.

HOW TO USE THIS BOOK

This book is a three-in-one resource. It is part educational resource, part guide, and part workbook to help you learn and take action in several different areas. I call this The Nourished Path™ to New Foods, the roadmap parents need to introduce their children to new food in positive and effective ways. The Nourished Path™ to New Foods starts with the basics. The stuff every parent of a picky eater should know. But it goes deeper, providing a systematic structure for those parents dealing with extreme picky eaters. Here's how this resource breaks down, and how you can get the most out of it:

Educational Resource: First, you'll learn why kids may be hesitant with new foods, including genetic links, learned behaviors, and everything in between. You'll understand how a broad range of foods may improve your child's overall health, and why this is a compelling reason to keep helping your child along the path of food acceptance.

Try New Food Guide: I'll teach you what it takes to set the stage for food introduction, and common sense strategies to help your child try and accept new foods without drama, threats, or meltdowns. Most importantly, you'll get handy tips (and cautions) to make sure you go about this in the most positive way possible, even if your child is a challenging eater. I will also give you tracking tools, feeding tips, motivational inspiration, and some nutritious food ideas along the way.

Workbook: Throughout the book, you'll have places to jot down your observations about your child and his eating. You'll have self-reflection exercises to complete. You'll have room to reflect on the tips and strategies you've tried and their outcomes—the good and the not so good. Not only will this workbook guide you along in helping your child, it will allow you to document the process. That way, when you have success, you'll be able to remember the details, and even return to them should you get side-tracked and need to retrace your efforts.

This book is for both boys and girls, and younger and older children. As such, I've tried to use both gender references, toggling between him and her. I've also used the terms picky eater, fussy eater, and selective eater interchangeably, mostly to satisfy those of you who prefer one term over the other.

Last, in my experience, there is almost never one strategy that converts your picky eater into a willing eater. On the contrary, it usually takes several strategies, used together and in complementary fashion, to see progress. I encourage you to use this workbook to the fullest. Document your thoughts, ideas, and feelings. Note where you are in this journey, including what you've learned about yourself and your child.

Whether you have a transitional picky eater (one who is going through a typical picky eating phase), a picky eater who has been stuck in the picky eating phase for quite a while (extreme picky eater), or you just want to help your new eater add foods to his diet in the most positive of ways (without creating a problem), there are certain principles and approaches that make the task a pleasant and productive experience for everyone.

In the end, my hope is that you will gain the knowledge, insight, and perspective you need to keep plugging along with adding new foods to your child's repertoire.

Let's get going!

CHAPTER 1

THE PICKY EATING CONTINUUM

From typical picky eater to extremely picky eater.

OST PARENTS I MEET ARE doing the best they can to raise kids who eat healthily. They have great hope and possibility in mind as they start solids with their baby. They dream about the exotic foods their child will eat—sushi, spicy foods, and all sorts of vegetables and whole grains. They imagine family vacations and dinners out where everyone eats together and food isn't a struggle. They visualize a happy and calm meal table.

Many of these same parents experience a very different reality, however. They have kids who are fickle and refuse to eat when something new is brought to the table; kids who like a particular food one day, then say they don't like it the next; kids who only eat certain foods; meltdowns over flecks of pepper in food, or foods touching each other on the plate; kids who cry at the table and ruin the meal; or kids who simply won't eat.

Whether your child is just becoming picky or stuck in the throes of extreme picky eating, you will want to learn about the basics of what I call the "picky eating continuum."

YOU CAN'T MAKE YOUR CHILD EAT

When my first child turned one year old, there was a lot going on. I was a clinical dietitian at Boston Children's Hospital and commuting 45 miles in and out of Boston each day. We had a daycare provider who closed her doors at 5:00 p.m. sharp. To say the stress of getting home on time was high is an understatement. By the time I rolled into daycare, I was hyped up and stressed out. My daughter felt that. We'd get home and I'd put her into the highchair for dinner. She wouldn't eat much.

Twenty-two years ago, I was (and still am) a follower of Ellyn Satter. I'd read *Child of Mine*, and was using the principles of the Division of Responsibility in Feeding with my daughter. When my girl indicated she was done eating, I ended the meal. Even though she was eating six times a day (snacks and meals), I didn't have a clue how much she was getting during the day. Yet, I knew she wasn't getting much with me. I had a nagging worry she wasn't getting enough. Her annual check-up confirmed this: she was riding along the 5th percentile for weight – the low end of the growth curve.

I was a pediatric dietitian with a child who wasn't growing well. Fear? Shame? Embarrassment? Check. Check. Check. I knew I'd be facing an even greater challenge. I was entering one of the toughest periods of childhood—Toddlerhood—a time when kids stop eating foods they like, eat a repetitive diet, and seem to exist on air.

Most parents know about picky eating, but the truth is, they aren't prepared for it. Not really. Some parents try to go with the flow, while others engage in the picky eating battle. They pull out all the tricks to get their child to try new food. They bribe their kids to eat their veggies or give in to food preferences by becoming short-order cooks. Some parents use a strong-arm approach, threatening and punishing their child to get them to eat or try something new.

Just as the saying goes, "You can lead a horse to water, but you cannot make him drink," the same holds true for kids. You can't make them eat. At least, not in a nurturing way. I knew I had to step back, assess, and revamp how I was managing nutrition and feeding. I had to look at my daughter's needs and look at myself.

Research tells us that adults who were picky eaters when they were younger still remember the negative interactions they experienced at the table.[5] I've heard this over and over from some of the parents I've worked with in the past. Meg remembers sitting at the dinner table when she was a child until nine o'clock at night. She couldn't get up until she ate her green beans. Karen got punished for stuffing peas down the radiator. Mary pushed food around her plate to make it look like she ate, while carefully tucking it under the rim of her plate. When caught, her father would yell at her and send her to her room for the night. I've heard other stories from parents who had to eat their dinner for breakfast the next day.

I'm hoping this book will prevent you from using these unproductive 'get my child to eat at all costs' tactics because you never know whether your child will take these strategies to heart or not. One thing I've learned over the years: It's difficult to develop a healthy relationship with food and an adventurous attitude about trying it while under pressure, stress, and fear. This is something I'll address further in Chapter Five. First, we need to explore the variable traits of the picky eater. Understanding this will help you identify where your child falls on the picky eating continuum.

THE TYPICAL PICKY EATER

Meet Isabella. She's three. She's a pretty good eater and has been all along. Here and there, she's refused food, but she always seems to welcome it back, eventually. Like the time she took a hiatus from yogurt, one of her regular breakfast and snack foods. At one point in time, Isabella couldn't seem to get enough yogurt, asking for it all the time. And then one day—poof!—she didn't want yogurt any more. She shook her head "no" when it was offered, and dodged the yogurt cup when it was put on her tray.

Her parents noticed she was less interested in yogurt, even refusing it, but they expected this to happen eventually, and decided not to make a big deal of it. Instead, they offered cottage cheese, other types of cheese, or milk with her meals to fill in the calcium gap. They introduced yogurt-based fruit smoothies, which Isabella loved, along with frozen yogurt and some baked items using yogurt, like muffins and quick breads.

One day at preschool, a snack of flavored yogurt was passed around. All the kids had some, and so did Isabella. The next day, Isabella asked for yogurt.

Isabella is a typical toddler eater. Liking food one day, then refusing it the next. Showing disinterest for a period of time, then warming back up and willingly integrating that food back into her diet.

It helped that her parents were adventurous themselves with food and cooking, as Isabella had been exposed to a number of different foods, ethnic dishes, and eating environments throughout her short childhood. While her parents couldn't avoid this picky eating phase, they sailed through it by knowing what to expect, keeping things positive (in other words, staying cool, calm and collected), and not pushing Isabella to eat what she did not want to eat.

> **FOOD FOR THOUGHT**
> Despite what appears to be 'not eating enough,' choosy children
> tend to stay at a healthy weight and grow well (often a surprising
> fact to parents!). Keep tabs on your child's growth chart to give
> you some peace of mind.

MY CHILD IS GETTING WORSE

Ten year old Sam is still picky with vegetables. His Mom and Dad have been waiting for him to turn a corner, but he won't touch them. They've tried everything, from slipping pureed veggies into casseroles, using tasty dips, and even summoning peer pressure at parties, but nothing's worked. In fact, they think they may have made things worse.

Even though picky eating is considered common for the toddler and preschool years, it can last longer, even getting worse when the wrong feeding techniques are used. Take my above example with Sam. His parents pressured him to eat and try new food. He resisted. When his parents used more pressure and other tricks, he pushed back and became even more resistant. This dynamic continued, worsening Sam's picky eating and facilitated a negative association with meal time.

Sam also learned that his refusal to eat often ended up in getting the food he really wanted to eat. This cycle persisted: Sam's negative behavior motivated his parents to fix the food he wanted, and his willingness to try new food dramatically declined.

Some strategies to get kids to eat seem like they will work, but they often backfire, making the situation worse. Translated: negative feeding interactions can prolong the picky eating phase, making it last longer than it needs to. We'll explore your feeding style and strategies later in Chapter Five, and how they may affect your child's willingness to eat, appetite regulation, and weight. It's pretty powerful stuff!

THE EXTREME PICKY EATER

Now I want to introduce you to Matthew. He is four—and he's pretty fussy about food. He is also in preschool. According to his parents, Matthew has been tough to feed his entire life. He was slow to establish nursing and didn't want to give it up when it was time to move on to eating the family food. He gagged on solid food and was a slow eater. He refused veggies from the very beginning, gagging on them. Fruit was better, but he preferred to eat it off a spoon, rather than touch it with his hands. From early on, Matthew seemed most at ease with dry cereal, crackers, and crunchy snacks.

Today, Matthew refuses many foods, and has a short list of items he will eat. Matthew's parents know he is lacking in vegetables and fruit, isn't getting enough protein (he won't eat meat and only drinks a bit of milk), and relies too heavily on carbs such as crackers, chips, and sweets.

When his parents add a new food to the meal, Matthew gets very upset. He cries or throws a tantrum, and refuses to eat. Just the other night, spaghetti, meatballs, and sauce served with a lettuce wedge sent him into a meltdown. These nights are hard on everyone. Frequently, Matthew's mom makes him something different to eat, which is usually plain noodles and chicken nuggets, or a bowl of cereal. She doesn't want him to be hungry or go to bed on an empty stomach. He is already too thin.

Over time, Matthew's "list" of liked foods got smaller and smaller. He was down to about twenty foods he would willingly eat. Knowing how limited his diet was, his parents were very worried about Matthew dropping another food from his diet. A common cold could change everything. Matthew could eliminate a food or two as a result, not to mention losing a few pounds, as well. His parents also suspected he was getting bored with his usual food routine, but they didn't know how to bring more variety to the table.

In my assessment, Matthew showed signs that he was more than "typically picky." His list of "liked" foods was shrinking, rather than expanding, and his emotional response to new foods was becoming more intense. Matthew demonstrated signs of extreme picky eating, also known as Avoidant Restrictive Food Intake Disorder (ARFID).

AVOIDANT RESTRICTIVE FOOD INTAKE DISORDER (ARFID)

Avoidant Restrictive Food Intake Disorder (ARFID) is characterized by a persistent disturbance in eating leading to weight loss or growth disturbances, nutrient deficiencies, dependence on supplements, and impaired psychosocial functioning. While typical picky eating signs are seen, ARFID tends to last longer and exhibits progressive limitations in food tolerance, food consumption, and nutrient intake.[6]

Experts categorize ARFID as an eating disorder, but it's not the same as anorexia, bulimia, or other known eating disorders. Those eating disorders are motivated by poor body image and a desire to reduce or change the weight, size, or shape of one's own body.

In the case of ARFID, selective eating is not motivated by weight concerns or body image. Children with ARFID are avoiding food because they fear it, or it's uncomfortable to eat. Not because they wish to lose weight. Obviously, with all this fear and discomfort around food and eating, anxiety is commonly part of the picture. In fact, it's estimated that 21% of children with ARFID also have anxiety and 58% have an anxiety disorder.[7] I'll discuss ARFID (extreme picky eating) in more detail in Chapter Nine.

> **DID YOU KNOW?**
> The resolution of extreme picky eating often requires professional help in the form of feeding therapy, nutrition intervention, family dynamic work, and psychological support for anxiety.

As you begin to use this workbook, I want you to have a good sense of your child's eating, in real time. If you're just starting out with feeding your child, I bet you have a willing eater. If you have a toddler, preschooler, or school-age child, you may be seeing some of the signs of picky eating. Whatever you're dealing with, you need to name it to address it. Use the reflection below to assess your child's eating, and in the next chapter you will be able to further identify the big picture.

REFLECTION:

Let's take a moment to assess your child's eating. Which type of eater do you have?

Check off the characteristics you see most often in your child.

Typical Picky Eater	Extreme Picky Eater
❏ Refuses food, especially veggies	❏ Refuses most new foods
❏ Rejects previously accepted food	❏ Eats food with similar textures
❏ Eats the same food, over and over	❏ Eats less than 20 different foods in the diet
❏ Refuses to try new food	❏ Eliminates major food groups
❏ Demonstrates fussiness with food	❏ Drops foods and doesn't regain them in the diet
❏ Shows disinterest in food	❏ Experiences anxiety or negative emotions with new food
❏ Eats limited variety or amounts of food	❏ Goes for days without eating
❏ Eats slowly	❏ Adds stress to mealtimes
❏ Has added some new foods to diet	❏ Eats different food from the family

CHAPTER 2

LOOKING AT THE WHOLE PICTURE

Your child's growth, eating habits, and feelings matter.

O NE OF THE FIRST THINGS I want to know when I'm working with families who are dealing with picky eating is how their child is growing. The second thing? What their child is eating. And the third, how their child is feeling about food and eating. In this chapter, we'll explore your child's growth, eating patterns, and behaviors around the table so that you have a good sense of the whole picture and a baseline for moving forward. This starting point will allow you to measure the progress for you and your child over time, while also framing your hopes.

HOW IS YOUR CHILD GROWING?

Growth is the hallmark of a well-nourished child. This is why pediatricians and dietitians like me always refer to a child's growth chart. Your child's growth chart is divided into a weight curve, a height curve, and a body mass index (BMI) curve. If you have a child under the age of two, you'll also see a head circumference curve.

The weight curve tells you how your child's weight compares to other children of the same age and gender. The height curve is similar: It tells you how tall your child is compared to other children with the same age and gender. The BMI chart is a calculated value using your child's weight and height. It represents your child's personal weight in relation to his height. This value is plotted on the BMI growth curve and compares your child's BMI to other children of the same age and gender. You can find growth chart resources in Appendix A.

Children and their weights and heights fall all over the growth curves. Some children are at the 5 percentile, some at the 75 percentile, and some will be at the 95 percentile. In other words, each child is different; and while these curves provide useful information, we have to be careful when using them as comparison norms among individual kids.

When evaluating a child's growth chart, I look for consistent progress along an established growth curve. In the case of picky eating, children can grow well or they can grow poorly. Some kids with a normal growth curve will not be well-nourished. For example, if a child isn't eating fruits and vegetables and not taking a daily multivitamin, he may *appear* to grow adequately, but he might also have a nutrient deficit. This is why it's important to look at eating patterns and food intake, as well.

The growth chart helps raise a red flag if a child is getting too much nutrition or too little. Increases in weight gain, or weight loss, and even a lack of weight gain can be seen on the growth chart, alerting me to a problem. Likewise, lack of height growth, or stunting, is also apparent on the curves. Although you may believe picky eaters are underweight, the truth is they run the gamut. Some are normal weight, some carry extra, unnecessary weight, and yes, some are underweight.

Of course, knowing what your child is routinely eating adds an important element to the picture. As I mentioned, kids can look like they are growing normally while getting inadequate nutrition. For example, your child can be missing calcium and vitamin D in his diet, yet still plug along on the growth chart. Certainly, when a child is tracking on his or her own personal, healthy growth trajectory, we can all breathe a little easier! However, when an established growth curve starts to change (up or down), we need to take a closer look.

REFLECTION:

Have you looked at your child's growth chart? If not, gather it from your pediatrician (it's an easy request through the portal or just a quick phone call request).

What do you notice about your child's weight curve? (steady growth, jumps up or down, etc.)

_____

_____

_____

What do you notice about your child's height curve?

_____

_____

_____

What do you notice about your child's BMI curve?

_____

_____

_____

After evaluating your child's growth chart, what stands out for you?

_____

_____

_____

WHAT IS YOUR CHILD REALLY EATING?

When your girlfriend brags about the pesto pasta her child ate, or the taco dinner her whole brood devoured, you may want to strangle her. Well, not really, but you know that feeling of frustration and inadequacy, right? You may also feel like your child will never be able to eat that way; that she'll never get there, no matter what you do.

I notice for many parents of picky eaters, it's easier to rattle off the foods their little one _won't_ eat instead of acknowledging the foods their child _will_ eat. I want to give some time and attention to a typical eating day for your child. List the foods your child typically eats on a normal day.

REFLECTION:

Mini-Food Diary: Take a moment to list the timing and foods your child eats on a typical day.

Time and Meal	Food and Drink (approximate amounts)

When you look at the foods your child is eating regularly, what is noteworthy (e.g. same foods, takes a long time to eat…)? What needs attention? What feelings do you experience when you look at this list?

_____

_____

_____

_____

_____

If your child is older, you may see foods that are your child's "go-to" items. You may also see eating patterns such as predictable times at which your child gets hungry, the usual location where your child likes to eat, and other habits your child has developed with his eating. You may also notice your child's favorite foods boldly represented in the mini-food diary. Perhaps they have a stronghold in her daily eating. Let's dig into that a bit.

Make a list of your child's favorite foods. These are the foods she asks for, and readily eats.

My child *likes to eat*...

_____	_____

You might be feeling frustrated with the foods your child likes to eat compared to the foods you *want* your child to eat. Coming to terms with your own frustrations can help you reset your mindset about helping your child try new foods.

Do you want your child to eat fish? Lasagna? Steak? Vegetables?

Fish is a healthy addition to any child's diet, but some parents aren't cooking it, or eating it themselves. Therefore, the exposure to fish is low, and so is the role modeling your child may need to see.

Lasagna is a combination dish with multiple ingredients, textures, and smells. In other words, lasagna is a complicated dish. As a result, kids may be timid around this food, as well as other casserole combinations. My own kids were not interested in lasagna until they were in their double digits.

Meat is certainly nutritious and loaded with nutrients, but it's also hard to chew. Some kids will quickly determine that meat is tough, too hard to chew, and doesn't feel safe.

And vegetables? They tend to be bitter, and may not have the eye appeal or odor some kids need to experience to be enticed to eat them.

Are there foods you wish your child would eat? List them here.

_____   _____

_____   _____

_____   _____

_____   _____

_____   _____

_____   _____

_____   _____

Why is it important your child eats these foods?

_____

_____

_____

_____

_____

_____

Aside from nutritional qualities, are there other reasons these foods should be eaten?

_____

_____

_____

_____

_____

_____

AN EXERCISE FOR PARENTS OF OLDER, PICKY EATERS

For the older child who has been fussy about food for a while, I want to explore some of the changes in foods that have happened over the years; especially the significant food preference changes. The point of this exercise is to explore any events or triggers that may have precipitated a change in your child's food preferences.

Let me clarify with a story. Amy is a mom to a 10-year-old boy. Jack has been selective with food for quite a while. To date, he has about thirty foods he will eat. When he was a toddler, he ate a wider variety of foods, especially in the fruit and vegetable category.

For example, Jack used to eat apple slices. When he started refusing them, Amy offered applesauce, which Jack accepted for a long time. Somewhere around first or second grade, Jack refused to eat applesauce. It would come back in his lunch box every day. Amy stopped packing it. Amy has always wondered why Jack stopped eating applesauce. Did something happen? Was he teased at school for bringing a pouch of applesauce? Did he get bored? Did he choke?

Jack's reason: "I just don't like it."

Last, let's make a list of foods your child *used to like and eat*. For example, my child used to eat _____, but isn't eating it now.

_____   _____

_____   _____

_____   _____

_____   _____

_____   _____

_____   _____

When you look at the foods your child used to eat, what are some of the circumstances surrounding his or her decision to drop this food? For example, a child may have gagged on a food, or she may have experienced anxiety around starting a new school or moving into a new home. She may have been teased, or punished for not eating enough of it.

The point of this exercise is to bring more awareness to the potential connection with the environment, your child's temperament, or other reasons behind dropping food from the diet. I'm not making excuses for your child's changing food preferences. On the contrary, I'm hoping to open your mind to the reasons your child may have dropped those foods he used to eat.

Used to Eat...	What happened?

YOUR FOOD GOALS

Now, let's look at your goals for your child's eating. You probably have foods you really want your child to eat. Foods you value for health reasons, foods you enjoy yourself, and foods the rest of the family enjoys.

Having a "wish list" of foods can be the basis of what you work on with your child. As you'll see later in the workbook, it's good to have goals around particular foods, but I always start with new foods that are quite similar to what your child is currently eating.

REFLECTION:

What "wish-list foods" do you value the most? List them below.

_____

_____

_____

_____

What would it be like if your child ate these foods?

_____

_____

_____

_____

What would happen if your child didn't eat these foods?

_____

_____

_____

_____

HOW IS YOUR CHILD FEELING?

Graham was always the last family member to come to the table. "I have to yell at him several times before he shows up," said his mom, Lori. "When he sits down, he's sullen, won't talk unless it's a complaint, and is generally very unhappy. Occasionally, he has a complete meltdown."

Your child's behavior around food and at the table is an important clue as to how he's dealing with food and eating. If he comes to the table curious, with a pleasant disposition and is a willing participant, you've got a good indication that your child is a happy eater. If he comes to the table reluctantly, has trouble sitting there, or seems agitated or unhappy, you've got clues that eating may be a stressor for him.

Of course, other things can disturb your child, but if you see that she is generally happy at the table, or generally unhappy, you can begin to uncover how the meal table environment influences her disposition.

In private, Graham told me that he felt like everyone was watching him eat. Not only did he receive comments about his eating from his parents, he got them from his siblings, as well. This amounted to a *perceived pressure to eat*, which almost immediately spiked his anxiety at meal times and made him more reluctant to come to the table. Eventually, it stole the joy from the community and connection of being together as a family.

It's true: A negative mealtime environment can overshadow a child's ability and willingness to eat. Alternatively, a positive, supportive environment can be just what a fussy eater needs to venture out and try new foods.

REFLECTION:

What does your mealtime environment look like? Check the boxes on either side that apply to the mealtime environment in your home.

Signs of a Positive Mealtime Environment	Signs of a Negative Mealtime Environment
☐ Parents are happy to have everyone around the table.	☐ Parents are easily annoyed by child's misbehavior or mistakes.
☐ Parents refrain from comments about the child's eating (good or bad).	☐ Parents comment about child's eating (too much, not enough, etc.)
☐ Parents don't talk about food or healthy eating.	☐ Parents lecture about healthy food, eating, and good health.
☐ Parents don't yell or threaten their child.	☐ Parents bribe, threaten, or punish child for not eating or for food choices.
☐ Parents model good manners.	☐ Parents don't fully partake in the menu offerings.
☐ Parents set an example of eating the foods served for mealtime.	☐ Parents ignore child's fullness or hunger, or they disregard child's food preferences.
☐ Parents are respectful of children's food preferences and appetite.	☐ Child doesn't want to come to the table.
☐ Child willingly comes to the table.	☐ Child complains about the menu.
☐ Child is curious about the menu.	☐ Child is fidgety, wants to leave the table.
☐ Child is calm.	☐ Child is defensive.
☐ Child is engaged in conversation.	☐ Child has outbursts or disruptive behavior at the table related to food.
☐ Child demonstrates manners.	☐ Child shows signs of anxiety or stress.

What do you notice about your mealtime environment?

_____

_____

_____

_____

What areas need more work?

_____

_____

_____

_____

What will you tackle as your first step towards a positive mealtime environment?

_____

_____

_____

_____

CHAPTER THREE

THE SCIENCE OF FOOD ACCEPTANCE

Kids aren't born liking food. They learn to like it, or not.

T HERE'S A LOT THAT GOES into liking food. First, a child needs to taste food, which means food needs to get on the tongue and taste buds. Then she needs to process the flavor through an integrated sensory system that includes all her senses: smell, appearance, touch, taste, and more.

If she decides the taste is pleasing, she may be willing to taste it again, and even grow to like it and eat it. If she decides she doesn't like the taste, she may refuse to try it again. Some kids won't get to the step of tasting new food. They'll simply smell or see a food and decide they don't like it. This can be very frustrating.

Tasting, eating, and liking new food is not always straightforward and simple. The good news? We have plenty of research that gives us hints about what works to encourage acceptance of new flavors and foods.

BLANK SLATE OR PRIMED PALATE?

I often hear people say babies are a "blank slate." Presumably, this means they have no knowledge or experience with the world around them. What and how they are exposed to the universe outside of the womb begins to shape their intellect, preferences, and perspective. However, this is not actually true for flavor preferences.

Babies experience flavors while they are growing in their mother's womb. Amniotic fluid is sweet, so babies are essentially "bathed in sweetness" during their gestation period. They also experience other maternal diet flavors. Many food flavors ingested by the mother during pregnancy are transferred to the baby through the amniotic fluid. For example, flavors from onion, garlic, tomato, broccoli, cauliflower, Thai food, and more can reach your baby.

Once born, if your baby was breastfed, she experienced the flavors of sweet and fat in your breast milk. Breast milk is naturally sweet and contains about 50% of the calories from fat. If you breastfed your child, sweet and fat flavors will be familiar to her and may influence flavor acceptance later on. While this may seem like a negative, it isn't. As I mentioned, other flavors from your diet such as onion and garlic are transmitted to your baby through your breast milk, too, priming her palate for these flavors later.

Research has shown that breastfed babies may be more accepting of a variety of flavors as they grow, and will be less picky.[8] This is due, in part, to the complex flavors they are exposed to in utero and through breast milk.

If your baby consumes infant formula, the flavor profile doesn't vary. This fact may make food introduction and acceptance a bit more challenging, so you'll have to be persistent in introducing a variety of flavors. By the time breastfed babies are starting solids, they already have some familiarity with flavors. Around six months of age, they begin to develop a salty flavor preference.[9]

You can offer a variety of foods to your baby through the first year of life, beginning at six months, when you begin introducing solid foods. Make a concerted effort to add a variety of flavors to her first foods, including spices and herbs. I cover how to do all of this in my book, *The Smart Mom's Guide to Starting Solids*.

> ### HOW TO USE FLAVOR IN FIRST FOODS
> - Add herbs: garlic, onion, cumin, basil, oregano, cinnamon, nutmeg
> - Use healthy fats: avocado, thinned nut butters*, olives, olive oil, ground seeds
> - Try aromatics: vinegar, citrus, spices
> - Spare the salt and sugar… a little bit goes a long way!

It is currently recommended to introduce age-appropriate peanuts and other nuts by age one.

For toddlers and older kids, keep in mind that introducing flavor remains paramount. Studies show that flavor and taste are primary drivers for eating. In other words, if food tastes good, kids will be more likely to try it, and even eat it, and perhaps learn to like it. Yet, despite this, I see parents fear flavor. They're afraid spicy food like salsa, garlic, or Indian cuisines will be "too much" for their child. There's no reason to fear flavor. Even if it's something you wouldn't choose to eat yourself, your child may enjoy it.

I believe a child will be more likely to eat food if it is flavorful. So, out with the bland food, and in with the spice, tang, and umami! In other words, keep flavor front and center. Here are a few ways to do so:

- Condiments can help a child try new food. Try barbeque sauce, steak sauce, salad dressings, hummus, guacamole, nut butter, sour cream, yogurt, and yes, ketchup.

- Embrace ethnic dishes such as Asian, Latin, French, and Indian dishes, which are full of exciting flavors.

- Vary the prep method for veggies: roasting brings out sweetness and stir-frying with herbs such as ginger can be a way to introduce new flavors.

REFLECTION:

Take a moment to reflect on your child's early experience with flavor.

What foods did you avoid and which ones did you include during pregnancy?

_____

_____

_____

_____

_____

What was your child's first experience with flavor (breast milk or formula)?

_____

_____

_____

_____

_____

What herbs, spices, or aromatics did you include in your baby's diet?

_____

_____

_____

_____

What has been your child's response to highly flavored food?

_____

_____

_____

_____

THE TASTE BUD FACTOR

Children experience flavors differently and this has to do with their taste buds. The average adult has about 10,000 taste buds, and it is said that children have more.[10] It's also believed that children have stronger and more intense taste buds, meaning they may experience flavor more strongly. For some kids, a little bit of flavor goes a long way. This intensity of flavor experience often shows up when kids try vegetables. Children may taste vegetables more strongly than adults, and find them more offensive to their taste buds.

As we age, our taste buds decrease in number, which is probably why older adults request saltier, sweeter foods. They experience a decrease in flavor intensity and they need *more* flavor to get the same flavor experience to which they've grown accustomed.

The notion that children will like all foods and eat them willingly at first bite is unrealistic. Of course, some children will taste something and like it immediately. This happens to adults too. However, when it comes to bitter, sour, or unusual flavors, many kids need to taste it more than once to appreciate and accept it.

Being born with a primed palate at birth provides a unique opportunity for you to build on and cultivate the flavors and textures in food you want to see your child eat. But you have to remember that this takes time. One of the most compelling reasons to introduce new food to your child early on is the idea of increasing your odds against a severely limited diet later on. The more foods your child can accumulate in his diet in the first two years, the better able he (and you) will be to withstand the picky eating stage when children naturally pare down their food variety and shorten their list of acceptable foods.

Every child will be different, and as we will explore later, *how* you introduce and support your child through food introduction will affect their rate of acceptance, as well. While some children will need a warm-up phase, you *should* be optimistic that your child can handle and accept new foods, according to his or her timetable.

Let's explore some of the other factors to consider as children learn to accept new foods, such as the sensory experience of food, the timing and age of introduction, blending flavors, and the influence of growth and appetite.

THE SENSORY EXPERIENCE OF FOOD

Children have their own sensory experiences. Some children may have heightened taste bud receptors for certain flavors (typically bitter or sweet) and thus experience these flavors more potently, as I mentioned above. They can experience flavors as highly offensive or highly attractive. We refer to these kids as supertasters (adults can be supertasters too).

Other children may be sensitive to the texture of food, or to its appearance, odor, or color. For example, some texture-sensitive kids shy away from wet, slippery foods like juicy fruits.

Others may dislike foods that are tough to chew, like cooked meats. Still others may steer clear of mushy foods like mashed potato or avocado.

Other kids are triggered by the odor of food, being offended by the smell of cooked eggs or cooked cruciferous vegetables like broccoli or cauliflower. Some kids just look at a food and determine they don't like what they see – the appearance of sliminess, dryness, or even sharp edges, for example.

FOOD IGNITES ALL THE SENSES

Food offers a sensory-focused experience for kids, mostly due to the senses that are triggered with the process of eating. Five senses are involved in the "experience" of food. They are taste, sight, touch, smell, and sound. Each sense has a special area in the brain where sensory signals are received and processed. Our sense organs are the ears, nose, mouth, skin, and eyes. Our bodies use our sensory organs to inform us of the surrounding environment so we can stay safe, communicate, and react.

For example, when your child sees asparagus, she may also smell it, touch it, and taste it. Her sensory organs start the transmission of information to the sensory areas of the brain, which ultimately get processed and lead to her overall "experience" of asparagus.

The Five Sensory Organs: ears, nose, mouth, skin, and eyes

The Five Senses: taste, sight, touch, smell, and sound

The Five Tastes: sweet, salt, sour, bitter, and umami

Let's focus a bit on the sense of taste. There are five basic tastes: sweet, salt, sour, bitter, and umami. Taste, for example, is received through the tongue, from taste buds and receptor cells on the tongue. Through this path, humans detect the chemicals that make up food.

Here are a few examples of each of these tastes and some of the foods that fall into their category:

Sweet: honey, maple syrup, cookies, candy, chocolate

Salt: soy sauce, salty crackers, chips, cheese, pickles

Sour: lemon, plain yogurt, cranberry juice (unsweetened), dill pickle

Bitter: arugula, celery, collard greens, broccoli, tomato

Umami: bacon, beef jerky, mushrooms, soy sauce, parmesan cheese

Children may react negatively to bitter and sour flavors by puckering their lips, gagging, shaking or shivering, or retracting from food. This is very normal and *does not* indicate whether your child likes a particular food or not. Demonstrating a "reaction" by drawing a facial expression is common when any new food is tried. Remember, multiple experiences are needed to warm up to a new food, especially bitter and sour flavors. Don't give up!

When your child tries sweet or salty foods, you may see a quick acceptance or liking of these foods. You may even see your child asking for more. While this can be disconcerting, especially when it's an "unhealthy" food, understand that this is natural because your child is already familiar with this taste.

Taste often gets confused with flavor. Let's clear this up: flavor is your sense of taste and smell *acting together* to form a perception of food. Taste and smell integrate to create the experience of flavor.

Although vegetables are naturally bitter, there are several ways you can minimize the bitterness and alter their taste to a more pleasing one. Cooking or roasting vegetables, or using flavor enhancers like fat, herbs, and spices can help mask the bitter taste and help your child warm up to them.

7 WAYS TO REDUCE THE BITTERNESS OF VEGETABLES

1. Roast them.

2. Saute them with healthy fats, like olive oil or canola oil.

3. Pair them with fruit, such as in a salad.

4. Dip them into salad dressing, hummus, or guacamole.

5. Blend them into a smoothie.

6. Blanch them to soften the flavor and the texture.

7. Cook with herbs, spices, or aromatics to alter the flavor.

Some children experience some or all of their senses more intensely. The noise of crunching (sound), the odor of food (smell), and the appearance of food (sight) may be intensely offensive, rendering a child unwilling or unable to eat. This experience can certainly overshadow the enjoyment of food and eating, contributing to prolonged picky eating.

Children who struggle with the sensory aspect of food may require more individualized help from a qualified nutrition or feeding professional. I'll address their specific needs later in Chapter Nine.

REFLECTION:

Does food and its characteristics turn your child off? If so, describe it below.

_____

_____

_____

_____

_____

INTEGRATING THE FIVE SENSES

Based on what I've described, it's clear that the experience around food and eating is not just about getting food on the tongue or taste buds. Experiencing food is about *all* the senses and the communication pathways in the brain that help kids make sense of what they are experiencing. This is called sensory integration.

For many parents, trying food means getting it on their child's tongue. But when we simply focus on getting our kids to taste food, we may disregard the importance of their other senses. In my experience, some children use a range of senses when it comes to food experiences. I've seen typically developing children, for example, especially young ones, become overwhelmed with the sensory experience and shut down. Or they may move more slowly to try new food than their parents would like. Still other children may enjoy (and embrace) the engagement of all the senses.

Children with a brain-based challenge such as ADHD, autism, or another neurological difference, may have difficulty integrating and processing all the sensory input that comes with food experiences. Remember those five areas of the brain? They must process all the data from the experience of food. In other words, each of the five senses needs to communicate with one another, or integrate, in order to interpret the experience of food. For some, this integration and processing step is where they get hung up.

For example, I've worked with children who shut down after looking at a food. They complain it appears too wet or too dry, and thus won't taste it. These kids do better with handling the food first, using the sense of touch. It's no surprise that I'm a big fan of allowing young children to fully experience food early on through simple things, such as allowing a child to douse himself in yogurt, smear food on his tray, and maintain a messy face while eating. Although these may seem counter-intuitive to good parenting, when you understand how important it is to fully embrace all the senses with eating, you can see how letting your child get messy may pay off in the future.

THE SUBTLE DIFFERENCE BETWEEN TASTING AND EATING

One misconception I hear from parents is the idea that tasting means chewing and swallowing. Let me clarify: Eating is tasting, chewing, and swallowing. Eating is *consuming* food. Conversely, tasting is engaging the tongue, taste buds, lips, and interior of the mouth, not necessarily chewing, and certainly not swallowing. Experiencing food can include looking at it, touching it, interacting with it, listening to it (as with someone eating it or hitting it on a table to demonstrate a food's hardness) and smelling it.

> **EATING VERSUS TASTING VERSUS EXPERIENCING FOOD**
>
> *Eating* is tasting, chewing, and swallowing food.
>
> *Tasting* is engaging the mouth, lips, tongue, and taste buds so they receive the chemicals that make up the taste of food.
>
> *Experiencing* food is seeing it, touching it, listening to it, smelling it, and tasting it.

It's important to understand the difference between tasting, eating, and experiencing food as we move forward. After all, this book is called *Try New Food*, not *Eat New Food*. When you know that your job is to help your child try or taste food, the temptation to use negative feeding practices (such as pressuring your child to eat more, take more bites, or make him sit at the table until he eats) disappears. Your compassion for and understanding of your child increases, which may translate to a more relaxed child; one who doesn't come to the table full of anxiety and worry.

TIMING OF FOOD INTRODUCTION & TEXTURE UPGRADES

Accepting new food is a process. Kids simply aren't born liking all foods. They must be repeatedly exposed to them in a positive, nurturing environment. Some kids will take to new food quickly, while others will need more time. And still others may never accept certain foods.

As parents, we are able to influence our child's food preferences. We can do this with what scientists call *repeated exposure*. Repeated exposure is simply offering your child a food over and over, in the context of a supportive environment.

For instance, you may be working on broccoli, a food with which many children struggle. To practice repeated exposure, for example, you might offer

Learning to Like Food

Variety

Repeated Exporsure

Food Acceptance

sautéed broccoli one night for dinner, cream of broccoli soup the following week, and some blanched broccoli and a dip a few days later. Your child continues to see broccoli as part of the menu and in different variations. In other words, your child is repeatedly exposed to broccoli.

Let's look at some of the scientific evidence on repeated exposure. I think this information will strengthen your resolve to use exposure strategically on this journey.

Researchers offered children a disliked vegetable eight subsequent times and saw an increased liking of it over time. And this vegetable acceptance lasted for years in most of the children. I call this "the magic of eight" exposures. The bottom line: repeatedly exposing young children to food they didn't like helped them overcome their dislike with lasting results.[11]

While the "magic of eight" is encouraging, the challenge is that many parents don't offer their child a rejected food more than once or twice. Why? Studies tell us they give up on offering foods their child rejects after about three or four food exposures.[12] Parents don't want to waste food, or bear the expense of uneaten food. They also find food rejection (and all the effort that goes into purchasing and preparing it) disheartening.

In my professional experience, it's hard to predict how many exposures a child may need to accept a new food. The research tells us that anywhere from 8 to 15, and even up to 50 exposures may be needed before a child will accept a new food in their diet.[13] The harsh reality is some children won't take a liking to certain foods, no matter how many times they are exposed to them.

Case in point, my husband has been exposed to mushrooms multiple times in his life. I can pretty much guarantee he will not touch them, let alone try to taste or eat them, even if I politely request him to do so. Yet, I've seen children who participate in food exposure therapy taste, eat, and add new foods to their repertoire when a methodical, repeated exposure approach is used. This is something I'll talk about later in the book.

Another interesting aspect about food acceptance involves the timing of starting solids and the food options you offer your baby. *When* you start solids may have an influence on his acceptance of foods, particularly vegetables. Not only that, the types and combinations of foods you offer can also set the stage for food preferences later on.

For example, one study looked at babies who were introduced to blends of vegetables (carrots, squash, and green peas) versus using the traditional approach of introducing a single veggie (carrots). The babies who received the veggie blend showed a greater acceptance of vegetables in general, and an increased likelihood of trying new food later on.[14]

Other studies have demonstrated that the more flavors and aromatics (translated: herbs and spices) babies experienced during the sensitive window for food acceptance (from 4 to 18 months), the more accepting they were of complex flavors later.[15]

I've worked with many picky eaters over the years; garden variety picky eaters (aka typical picky eaters) and more extreme cases. I've noticed that kids who start late with solids, or those who are slow to transition to more texture in their diet tend to be more selective compared to their same-age peers.

Not surprisingly, we have research that backs this up too. In one study, kids who were still on pureed, smooth foods at age 9 months were more likely to be picky at age 7 years than those kids who advanced through textures age appropriately.[16]

While it's hard to know if failing to start solids on time or at a slower progression along the texture spectrum will lead to resistance around trying new food, we do know that delays in food introduction and texture upgrades may signal eating trouble in the future.

What can you do? Pay attention to starting solids on time (around six months), be diligent with food variety, hit the texture upgrades in a timely manner, and get curious about any delays or challenges with eating you see. My book, *The Smart Mom's Guide to Starting Solids* can help you through this transition. And if you're well past this stage, don't worry, you can still help your child. Keep reading and working through this workbook.

THE RISE AND FALL OF THE HONEYMOON PHASE OF FEEDING

Sarah loved feeding her baby. Her girl would eat anything Sarah gave her. Sure, sometimes she grimaced, especially when Sarah gave her a new vegetable. But Sarah knew this was a natural response because veggies were bitter. She didn't let funny faces from her little girl deter her from offering lots of different flavors.

Research tells us that babies are most sensitive and receptive to flavors in their diet between the ages of 4 and 18 months, but particularly so between 4 and 6 months.[14] This is a point of confusion for many parents because public health recommendations are to delay solid food introduction until 6 months. The reason for the "wait until 6 months" advice is to prevent food allergy, problematic weight status, choking, and more.

During the first year of life when every food is a brand new food for your baby, feeding is often enjoyable for both you and your child. My *Fearless Feeding* co-author and I call this the *honeymoon phase of feeding*. It's a time when babies are willing recipients of almost any food and flavor you offer.

Parents love this phase of feeding because it's so rewarding. You begin starting solids and you hesitantly offer your baby sweet potatoes. She gobbles it up. With more confidence, you try green beans, then squash, and your baby happily eats it all. This is a blast! Soon, you are exploring all types of food, from new flavors to more complex flavor combinations, and you're having success. It feels *great*.

The honeymoon phase is rewarding, positive, and pleasing for several reasons. For one, your baby is in that sensitive period where she is accepting of new tastes and experiences. Not only is she learning about flavor and texture, she is learning to engage and communicate with you through feeding. She also has high nutritional needs and an appetite that goes with it. In other words, she's hungry and this makes her want to eat.

When toddlerhood hits, the honeymoon for many parents (and kids) starts to dwindle and end. Toddlers become less willing to try new food and accept new flavors for a variety of reasons. Developmentally, it's their job to separate from you and become more independent. Simultaneously, toddlers thrive on routine and want control. This may translate to "no," or food refusal, a demand for independence, such as "I do it," and repetition in many areas of their lives, including food. Simply stated, their developmental stage changes their motivation and this shows up in their eating.

Toddlers also experience a slowing in their growth. Their daily calorie requirement based on their weight decreases too. They simply don't require as many calories per pound of body weight compared to that first year of life. With slowed growth and reduced caloric needs, you can imagine that appetite follows. Yes, appetite takes a nosedive. Don't get me wrong. Toddlers still have an appetite, but it becomes fickle and unpredictable.

Toddlers still need a nutrient-rich diet to support the optimal growth of their body and brain. Food selection remains important. (We'll dig into food and nutrition in the next chapter.) Unfortunately, some toddlers get exposed to the flavors of sugar, fat, and salt on a regular basis which may encourage strong preferences for these flavors.

Based on everything that's going on with toddlers, it should be no surprise they begin to get a bit repetitive in their food preferences. They may want to eat certain foods day after day, and this tends to be the familiar foods they like. This is a food jag, mentioned in Chapter One.

As you hear all these changes in toddlerhood, you may think it's a good idea to ask your toddler what he wants to eat. After all, why waste effort and food? I would advise you avoid asking your toddler the question, "What do you want to eat?" Why? Your toddler will tell you what they know and like to eat. She won't branch out, be adventurous, and suggest something new. Toddlers don't have the mental acuity to know of a new food suggestion, nor are they developmentally driven to do this.

REFLECTION:

What "typical" toddler behaviors do you see in your child?

_____

_____

_____

_____

_____

_____

_____

_____

_____

Overall, during toddlerhood that window of opportunity for food acceptance begins to close. In other words, the honeymoon phase ends and the work begins. The good news? With a bit of strategy, patience, and fun, you can encourage your child to try new food while developing a healthy relationship with it.

As your child grows up and enters school, the influence of peers, other grownups, and activities may naturally open your child up to experimenting with and accepting new flavors and foods. Many picky eaters turn the corner during the school years. This is a time to engage your child in food activities, something I explore further in Chapter Eight. If your child doesn't show increasing interest in food, or is getting worse, he may need more professional help, something I give you guidance about in Chapter Nine.

I think we can agree that all children need to learn to accept new foods. Some will do it with ease. Others go through phases where adding new foods is more challenging. And still others will have a hard time accumulating new foods, no matter what you do.

How do you know if your child is getting the food and nutrients he needs? How do you optimize the day-to-day diet while strategizing which new foods to work on? Don't worry. We are addressing food and nutrients next. I want you to have a good sense of nutrition, so you can worry less as you move forward with helping your child try new foods.

CHAPTER FOUR

ALL ABOUT FOOD: NUTRIENTS, VARIETY & BALANCE

Nobody has an ideal diet. Yet, we can all work towards one.

THE PERFECT DIET. AH, YES, there's so much stigma, idealism and guilt surrounding this concept. For the most part, the perfect diet is elusive for most of us. Even me. At one end, people are far from the ideal, eating a diet full of sugar, processed, and nutritionally empty food. At the other end, people are obsessed with local, organic, dairy-free, gluten-free, fresh food from the earth…and possibly creating more hang-ups for themselves and their families.

I've always been a believer in moderation when it comes to food. Everything can fit as long as you don't go overboard. That means there is room for sweets and treats, while carbs, dairy, and grains can have a place on the plate as well. It's all about balance.

In this chapter, I will dig into some simple, practical approaches to getting a healthy diet on board for your child. I take a simple, uncomplicated approach. After all, if your child isn't willing to try new food, why get hung up on the "perfect diet"? While you may not be where you want to be with nutrition yet, I want you to have some basic nutrition goals in mind as you set out to help your child try new food.

THE IMPORTANCE OF FOOD SELECTION

As I shared with you in the introduction of this book, I made a big mistake with my first child. I failed to keep my eye on the nutritional balance of her diet. As a result, she became anemic. Unfortunately, many healthcare providers today don't want to look at or acknowledge the real concern of nutrition for young, growing children. They will tell you to not worry about what your child is eating. They'll encourage you to focus on feeding and the relationship that forms during this interaction with your child. They'll tell you that food and nutrients will work themselves out without much intervention from you.

Often it will. But sometimes it won't. Like in my case.

When you hear messages that food and nutrients don't matter much, you pay less attention—or perhaps no attention—to your child's food balance, variety, and potential nutrient gaps. And that can be disastrous for your child. I'm not suggesting you be obsessive about food. But I do think you should be aware of the basics, enough so that if your child is missing out in certain areas of his diet, you know what to do. Or at a minimum, that it needs to be addressed.

In my work with children, I've seen several incidences of nutrient deficiencies, growth failure, and repeated illnesses in kids who don't get the nutrition they need. I'll highlight a few, because these cases altered the way I think about food and nutrients for all children. My own personal experience and my experiences with families over the years have formed my approach on nourishing the whole child with food and feeding, and an eye on development.

One case I cannot forget is the mother who decided that iron-fortified cereal was toxic for her baby, so she avoided it. As her child got older, he became typically picky and wouldn't eat meat or veggies. Mom was suspicious of vitamin and mineral supplements, so she steered clear of them. (Thank you, anti-vaccination and anti-medication celebrities!) Around the age of three or four, she noticed her son had developed tics. (Tics are a habitual contraction of a muscle, most commonly in the face.) After many doctor visits and evaluations, there was no conclusion for the etiology of her son's tics. Her neurologist shared that he felt the tics were probably related to poor iron intake from an early age.

> The latest evidence suggests that iron deficiency anemia is increasing in prevalence for children. Up to 20% of kids are anemic due to an iron deficiency in their diet.[17]

Another memorable case involves an older child who was a picky eater and an athlete. He was referred to me after several bone fractures occurred in one year. After looking at his usual diet, it was clear milk, dairy products and dairy alternatives were not part of his nutrition plan, not to mention he wasn't successfully meeting his energy or protein needs. More importantly, there had been no supplementation to address his dietary deficits. In his case, the lack of calcium and vitamin D made his bones weak and prone to fractures.

In the scientific literature, we have evidence that rickets and scurvy are making a comeback.[18,][19] Rickets is a bone disease due to inadequate vitamin D in the diet (and from sun exposure). Bones need vitamin D to let calcium in so they become dense and hard. When vitamin D is inadequate, the bones don't harden sufficiently, and instead remain soft. As children grow, the long bones of the legs may bow out, resulting in a bow-legged appearance.

Scurvy is the result of a vitamin C deficiency. We are starting to see this in extreme picky eaters who don't eat fruit and aren't supplemented with the vitamin. Scurvy is characterized by anemia, exhaustion, spontaneous bleeding, pain in the limbs, especially the legs, and sometimes ulceration of the gums. Scurvy can be quite debilitating.

Food and nutrients matter, my friend. So does the feeding relationship. I believe it's an equal partnership. I'll dig into feeding in depth in the next chapter. But the nugget for you is: you need to pay attention to both.

THE NEED FOR NUTRIENT-RICH FOODS

The "food doesn't matter" message can be a misleading one, undermining your success at keeping your child healthy and well-nourished. And, it counteracts everything we know about the first 1,000 days of life (the period between conception to age two years).

During the first 1,000 days, the brain and body are developing like no other time in life. While calories help the body grow, they're not enough for the brain to optimally develop. All nutrients are needed for brain growth but some are particularly important in supporting brain development. They include protein, zinc, iron, choline, folate, iodine, vitamins A, D, B6, and B12, and long-chain polyunsaturated fatty acids.

When babies don't receive this complement of nutrients, deficits in brain development including intelligence and mental health can occur. These disturbances can last a lifetime. In addition, what expectant mothers and their young babies eat molds their future health, particularly of the heart, the potential for diabetes, and problematic body weight.

Additionally, young children have tiny tummies. This fact prevents them from eating large meals. In turn, we have to be conscious of smaller meals that pack a nutritional punch. Older children need good nutrition so they pay attention and learn in the school setting. Distractibility, literacy, and memory are all influenced by nutrients from your child's diet.

So, in my professional opinion, nutrients and food *do* matter. Quite a bit. Whether or not you have a baby, a toddler, or an older child, nutrients are important for all kids. Check the Appendix for a short list of food sources. While it's not a complete list, it will help you target nutrient-rich food sources for your child. You can find more extensive food and nutrient lists in *Fearless Feeding*.

HEALTHY FOOD VARIETY AND BALANCE

Your child gets nutrients from food or from a supplement. Ideally, food is your first source for nutrients. Not only does food contain important ones for growth and development, it has other "ingredients" like phytochemicals, fiber, probiotics, and flavonoids which enhance their effect on your child's health. You can't package these elements in a pill or gummy supplement. I promote a food first philosophy as the primary source of nutrients for all children.

Yet, if you're dealing with a picky eater, this variety and balance message may seem far-fetched. Bear with me. I want you to have a sense of the nutrient-rich diet for which you are striving. Hence, I'm going to take you through a few basic child nutrition concepts.

I believe the best way for children to get a vast array of nutrients is through offering a variety of different foods. We have an icon and guideline called *MyPlate* (located at https://www.choosemyplate.gov/) and it's a useful resource for selecting a variety of different foods for your child. *MyPlate* divides food into categories, or food groups.

They are:

Protein: eggs, lean meats, fish, beans, nuts (also part of the fats group), tofu, and other soy products

Dairy: milk and milk products like yogurt and cheese

Fruit: fresh, canned, frozen, and 100% juices

Vegetables: fresh, canned, frozen, and 100% juices

Grains: bread, crackers, cereals, pasta, rice, and other products made from grains

Fats/Oils: plant-based oils like olive and canola oil, avocado, nuts, and seeds

I include one additional group called Fun Foods.

Fun Foods: sweets like candy, sugar-sweetened beverages, cake, cookies, and other desserts; and high fat foods like French fries and fried calamari

The *MyPlate* food groups target important, specific nutrients.

For example, the fruit group and vegetable group target potassium, vitamins A and C, and fiber, among other nutrients. The protein group covers iron, zinc, vitamin B12 and more. The dairy group covers calcium, vitamin D, and potassium. I could go on and on, but you get the picture.

The more food groups you include in your child's meals and snacks, the better chance he has to get an optimal variety of nutrients.

The Nutrients from Food Groups	
Protein Group	Iron, zinc, B vitamins (niacin, thiamin, riboflavin, and B6), vitamin E, magnesium
Grain Group	Fiber, B vitamins (thiamin, riboflavin, niacin, and folate), iron, magnesium, and selenium
Fruit Group	Vitamin C, fiber, potassium, folate
Vegetable Group	Vitamin A, vitamin C, fiber, potassium, folate
Dairy Group	Calcium, vitamin D, potassium, protein
Healthy Fats or Oils Group	Vitamin E, DHA, omega-3 fatty acids

Note: adapted from www.MyPlate.gov

A BALANCED PLATE FOR MEALS AND SNACKS

A balanced meal plan is important for growing children. First, offering different foods as outlined in the picture below increases the chance your child will receive the majority of his nutritional requirements for growth. Second, the timing of meals and snacks helps cover your child's hunger and appetite so that she is better able to come to the table hungry and regulate her eating. In the end, a balanced meal plan helps your child meet nutritional requirements, while eating in a more intuitive manner (for hunger and appetite, rather than boredom or other outside triggers).

Here's a way I set up a balanced meal plan using the basic food groups. Start with protein first. Protein is important for growth and for appetite control, so I like to see it take a starring role at meals and most snacks. The protein food can be beef, poultry, fish, eggs, and beans, or it can be something from the dairy group (also a good source of protein) like milk or yogurt.

Second, pick fruit and vegetables. Yes, I like to see fruit on the table at all major meals. It takes the pressure off eating veggies if you have a picky eater, and it's a great source of nutrients. If your child has a sweet tooth, it's a good substitute for dessert.

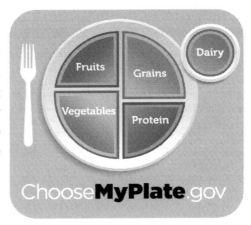

Last, fill in the meal plan with (whole) grains and dairy (if it hasn't been added yet). Most of the time, incorporate whole grains, or those grains that haven't lost their fiber content due to processing or refining. Thankfully, you can purchase white whole wheat or white whole grain pasta for children who refuse traditional whole grain bread and pasta.

THREE SIMPLE STEPS TO PLANNING A BALANCED MEAL

1. Choose a protein-based food.

2. Pick a fruit and/or a vegetable. Do both if you can!

3. Balance the meal with whole grains and a dairy source (if you haven't done so already).

You may be experiencing a different reality when it comes to a balanced plate: Your child's plate may not look balanced at all. That's okay. You (and your child) will get there. When your child has transitioned to using a plate (rather than eating off the highchair tray or table top), make sure to keep that routine in place. One thing I see happening in families with picky eaters is there may not be a plate for the child because he is eating separate meals and coming to the table with food in hand. Make the effort to normalize the meal plate as much as possible. Some families with picky eaters are out of the habit of sitting at a table with a plate, cup, and utensils. Set a place and plate for your child. Use utensils at his place setting. Arrange meal items on the plate, even if there may be limited variety and amounts of food. This routine will solidify the structure of mealtime and help normalize a balanced plate.

WHERE DO FUN FOODS FIT?

Nourishing foods, or those nutritious foods your child should be eating daily, are different from Fun Foods. Fun Foods are nutrient-poor, calorie-rich foods like candy, soda, cookies, cake, pie, and fried foods. I use a simple food "rule" to help parents and kids fit Fun Foods into the diet without tipping the balance to the unhealthy side. I call it the 90/10 Rule.

The 90/10 Rule makes it easy to sift through foods, categorize them, and decide which Fun Foods to eat, and when to eat them. Food balance can be easily achieved, resulting in a healthy diet that maximizes nourishing foods and moderates the less nutritious, indulgent ones.

Here's how the 90/10 Rule breaks down:

- 90% of your child's food consumption during the day should come from nourishing foods, or those food groups detailed above.

- 10% of what your child eats during the day, on average, may come from Fun Foods. For most healthy children, this ends up being 1 or 2 Fun Foods, in a normal or regular portion size, on average, each day.

Balancing Fun Food with a diet full of nutritious food is really the key to healthy eating. It's the best of both worlds — balanced, nutritious food for growth, development, and health, plus indulgent food to satisfy desire and help children learn to navigate these foods in their diet.

Some parents of fussy eaters tell me their children love Fun Foods and they have more difficulty getting their child to eat other, more nutritious foods. They tell me their child exceeds the

10% Fun Food goal, by a considerable amount. If this is the case for you, try the 90/10 Rule. It can be a gradual way out of this predicament. Start with where you are now (30% Fun Food or 25% Fun Food, for example), and strive to cut back a little bit at a time. Remember, your goal is 10%, but any reduction in Fun Food is a good accomplishment!

HOW OFTEN SHOULD MEALS AND SNACKS OCCUR?

The timing of a balanced meal plan matters too. In fact, the timing of meals and snacks can work for you, or against you. Get the timing right, and your child will be satisfied after eating, and less likely to ask for more food afterward. Get the timing wrong and your child will be hungry, asking for snacks, and potentially grazing with or without your permission.

I base my meal timing recommendations on basic physiology. A child's tummy fills up and empties faster than an adult's. This is primarily due to it being smaller. Because of the smaller size, children need to eat more frequently.

For instance, a toddler has a very little tummy, so I recommend setting up meal timing every two to three hours. Translated: a meal or snack should be scheduled every two-to-three hours throughout the day. This provides six eating opportunities each day and will help meet nutritional needs while covering hunger and appetite.

Example (toddler): Breakfast at 6 am; Snack at 9 am; Lunch at 11:30 am; Snack at 2 pm; Dinner at 5 pm; Snack at 7 pm

The school-age child should have a meal plan that reflects a three- to four-hour window between meals and snacks. The teen does well with meal timing scheduled every three-to-five hours, depending on growth spurt, activities, and overall daily life events.

Example (child): Breakfast at 7 am; Snack at 9:30 am; Lunch at 12:30 pm; Snack at 3:30 pm; Dinner at 7 pm

I think meal timing is critical to helping your child regulate his eating. In other words, helping him eat the right amount of foods to satisfy his appetite. I see kids go too long without eating and experience the sensation of being overly hungry. You know where that can lead: A greater likelihood of overeating unhealthy foods. Or, I see the child who grazes and snacks frequently throughout the day. This child may get too much food and may never feel hungry. Meal timing (and the supportive kitchen boundaries you need to back you up) can help tame those eating extremes.

DO PORTION SIZES MATTER?

Food portions for kids are smaller than they are for adults. No brainer, right? If you think about the size of a child compared to an adult, it makes sense that children would need smaller food portions. Yet studies show that some parents serve their children amounts of food more in line with a full-grown adult.[20]

Knowing the norm for a child-size portion will help you not only target the right amount of food to begin with, it will help you avoid overfeeding (and overwhelming) your child.

I go against the grain when it comes to food portions for kids. I like to use the concept of a "starter portion." This is an amount of food with which to start. After that, allow your child's appetite to guide how much she eats. I also think it's best to start small and "go big" later. Let your child ask for more, rather than start with overzealous goals and big portions, which can be overwhelming to your child, especially if he's finicky about food.

Instead, the goal is to help your child feel comfortable, with no intimidation. You can do this by using a very small amount, or small portion, of a new food. Even though we have accepted portion sizes for children, for the picky eater, these portions may be too big. You may want to try a half portion or smaller, or go even smaller than that if you have a very picky eater.

For instance, use a tablespoon, teaspoon or even less. Again, the goal is to create confidence and capability with the amount of food you present. Your child can always have more if desired.

Using a "starter portion" approach teaches a reference for reasonable portions of food and allows your child to visualize age-appropriate food amounts. While offering "starter portions" will build awareness, it is not license to restrict or control your child's food intake.

Here's a quick reference to some household items that correspond with portions. Be sure to check the table in the Appendix for a more descriptive portion guide for kids.

- a deck of cards for meat or fish

- 3 dice for cheese

- a lightbulb for rice and pasta

- a baseball for fruits/veggies, milk, and breakfast cereals

- a poker chip for oils, salad dressings, and other fats

- a hockey puck for biscuits and muffins

- a CD for waffles and pancakes

Your child should be allowed to eat an array of food groups at mealtime, in amounts that satisfy her appetite. Starter portions are simply a place to begin with food offerings.

REFLECTION:

Take a moment to absorb the principles of a healthy diet and reflect upon the areas where you are succeeding and which areas need more attention.

Which food groups does your child eat well?

_____

_____

_____

What food groups may be missing for your child?

_____

_____

_____

As an extension of these, which nutrients concern you the most?

_____

_____

_____

Which areas (variety, balance, portions) need more work?

_____

_____

_____

What is your first step for improving your child's diet?

_____

_____

_____

PUTTING IT ALL TOGETHER

Giving your child the best nutrition you can is the goal, even if your child is eating a limited variety of foods. A balanced meal plan includes a variety of food groups so the key nutrients for growth and development are met each day (or at least on average over the course of a week). If you're not there yet, that's ok! This gives you a goal and a framework to work towards. You'll still want to include those food groups that your child might be shunning. Don't worry, I'll give you some options for how to do that later in this workbook.

Use starter portions, and optimize meal timing based on your child's age to better match your child's appetite. I want your child to come to the table hungry. Using balance, variety, and portions—a three-pronged method—you can create a healthy diet for your child, while teaching him how to balance food and regulate his eating.

If you're not having success with certain food groups, a supplement to fill the nutrient gaps may be needed.

WHEN YOUR CHILD ISN'T GETTING THE FOOD HE NEEDS

Some kids do not get the myriad of nutrients they need from food, particularly if they are super selective and avoid entire food groups. In this instance, a supplement may be warranted.

If you notice a repetitive pattern of inadequate food groups or nutrients, you'll want to seek out a supplement. For example, if your child won't eat *any* fish, an omega-3 supplement will be in order. If he doesn't like milk or is unable to drink it (food allergy), sourcing a calcium and vitamin D supplement is prudent. If she doesn't like meat, and you aren't having success with finding alternative iron- and zinc-based food sources that she *will* eat, you'll want to consider a multivitamin and mineral supplement with iron and zinc.

Oftentimes, an age-appropriate multivitamin and mineral supplement will offer many of the vitamins and minerals found in fruits and vegetables, plus other important nutrients like vitamin D, iron, and zinc.

One nutrient that falls short in a supplement is calcium. If your child is not consuming milk, dairy products, or fortified dairy substitutes regularly, you'll want to discuss a calcium source for your child with a dietitian or doctor.

I've included some of my favorite vitamin and mineral supplements in the Appendix.

If your child isn't growing well, it's fair to assume he's missing out on sufficient calories and nutrients. In this case, a supplemental beverage that can supply micronutrients, minerals, and a source of calories and protein may be needed. Check the Appendix for examples of commercial drinks and some homemade versions.

CHAPTER FIVE

YOUR CHILD, YOU & NEW FOOD
Your child is unique and so are you.

EACH KID IS DIFFERENT. YES, I know. This phrase is a little bit cliché, but there's a lot of truth to it. Here's the thing: You are unique, too. The melding of you and your child around food and eating can be a pleasant synergy or a constant clash of wills. Throw in your past experiences of being fed as a child and we've got a potpourri of "stuff" to think about and work through.

Creating positive experiences with food is so critical! It all begins at the table. Many experts in the area of feeding and food introduction believe the feeding environment must be pressure-free and full of love, patience, and a nurturing spirit. I happen to be one of those experts. Your child must have a positive experience with food and eating whether he falls on the picky eating spectrum or not.

Not only that, but your child's developmental stage and temperament are undeniable pieces of the puzzle too. Understanding this is a powerful ally in helping your child try new food. Are you ready to learn more?

YOUR FEEDING STYLE

I don't think I'll ever be able to write a book that doesn't somehow weave in the topic of feeding. Feeding is *always* part of the childhood nutrition conversation for me. I include the topic in everything I do, from my childhood nutrition "bible," *Fearless Feeding,* and online educational programs to the other books, articles, and podcasts on my website. In this chapter, we are going to take a deep dive into the feeding styles and practices that are part of your daily routine and try to figure out if they are helpful, or getting in the way.

Ellyn Satter coined the term *feeding relationship* and defines it as:

> *"The complex of interactions that takes place between parent and child as*
> *they engage in food selection, ingestion, and regulation behaviors."* [21]

A parent who is successful with feeding:

- Trusts and depends on information coming from the child about timing, amount, preference, pacing, and eating capability.

- Supports a child's developmental tasks and helps the child develop positive attitudes about self and the world.

- Recognizes feeding cues and responds appropriately to them.

- Enhances the child's ability to consume a nutritionally adequate diet and to regulate appropriately the quantity eaten.

The feeding relationship develops between you and your child over time and reflects your feeding style, daily feeding practices, your child's temperament, and developmental stage. We know early on, a healthy feeding relationship is integral to the trust, security and predictability a child will come to rely on as he grows up.

As you'll learn, your daily feeding interactions are important in helping your child learn and thrive with food. Thus, while food is the backbone of health, feeding is the foundation of a healthy relationship with food, body, and self. In other words, food and feeding are *equally* important. If you want to raise a child who tries new food, you'll want to pay equal attention to positive feeding.

To that end, let's break down what we know about feeding styles here. There are four feeding styles documented in the scientific literature. The names of each have changed over the years, but these are the latest descriptors:

CONTROLLING FEEDING STYLE

The controlling feeding style is "parent-centered." This feeding style emphasizes rules around eating, including trying new foods and completing a meal. Eating is directed by the parent, rather than self-directed by the child. For example, dessert may be contingent on eating dinner. Parents may plate food for their children. When kids are raised with this feeding style, they may become resistant to trying new food, get pickier, or overeat. Weight problems, both underweight and overweight, are correlated with this feeding style.[22]

INDULGENT FEEDING STYLE

This style is a child-directed feeding style, and is characterized by a parent who is more inclined to say yes to food requests, who has loose structure around feeding, and few limits around food. Even though the parent says "no" or a limitation is given, ultimately the child receives what she wants. Children of parents with an indulgent feeding style may be more likely to gain unnecessary weight, be out of touch with their hunger and fullness, and eat more calorie-dense foods.[23]

UNINVOLVED FEEDING STYLE

With this feeding style, food and eating are less important for the parent, and that may show up in feeding. For example, planning for meals, shopping for food, and regular meal times may be erratic and unpredictable. Children, in turn, may feel insecure about food, unsure about when they will have their next meal, whether they will like it, and if it will be enough. These kids may have a scarcity mindset around food, be more focused on or triggered by it, and frequently question the details around mealtime.[24]

DIPLOMATIC OR LOVE WITH LIMITS FEEDING STYLE

The best and most productive feeding style is the "love with limits" style, which promotes structure with meals and snacks, sets limits around them, and promotes independent thinking and self-regulation. For example, diplomatic feeders determine the details around the meal (what will be served, when it will happen, and where it will be served), but allow the child to decide whether and how much to eat from what is available. Trust and boundaries are the basis of this parent feeding style. Children who are raised this way tend to be leaner, good at self-regulating their food consumption, and feel secure about food and eating. The most current research advocates this style of feeding as an effective way to raise healthy kids who know how to regulate their appetite, and learn to eat a variety of foods.[25]

Of course, you do not use one feeding style all of the time. It's natural to use bits and pieces of one style or another. For instance, when you see your child overindulging on sweets at a party, you may become more controlling. When you're stressed and busy, you may allow treats more liberally, or fail to plan meals as you usually would.

Despite your tendency to flirt with all the feeding styles, you do have one that is used the most. This feeding style often reflects how you were fed as a child and can be a direct extension:

Your parents were controlling with feeding and you are, too. Or, you may be using a different one on purpose: Your parents were indulgent, and you've taken a different approach.

Your feeding style, nonetheless, is deeply ingrained and influences how you feed your own kids. And, if it's one of the negative feeding styles (controlling, indulgent or uninvolved), it may be getting in the way of your success with helping your child try new food.

REFLECTION:

What memories do you have about mealtimes from your childhood? Are they positive or negative?

_____

_____

_____

_____

What similarities with your parents' feeding style and yourself do you see?

_____

_____

_____

_____

How are you different with feeding than what you remember about your parents' style?

_____

_____

_____

_____

How does your partner's childhood feeding history influence your mealtime?

_____

_____

_____

_____

YOUR DAILY FEEDING TACTICS

One of the easiest ways to figure out which feeding style you use the most is to take a look at your day-to-day feeding tactics. In the research, these are called _feeding practices_. Some of the most detrimental feeding practices for any child include pressure to eat, short-order cooking, and using food as a reward. These can be particularly problematic for picky eaters. Let's take a look at each one.

PRESSURE TO EAT

Pressure to eat is one of the most common feeding practices I see parents use when interacting with their kids around the meal table. From "*Just try it!*" to "*Two more bites before you can get down,*" pressure comes in many forms. For example, begging or pleading with your child to take another bite, or to try a new food; evaluating how well or how poorly your child has eaten; threats or consequences for not eating a certain food or not eating enough; taking away privileges or food as a result of what or how much your child has eaten; and even jubilant cries of success and praise for trying a new food.

Yes, even positive strokes can feel like pressure to a child. Using pressure to motivate your child's eating is simply not motivating. In fact, according to research, it can induce early fullness, and contribute to more pickiness.[26]

This happened to Will, a five-year-old boy I worked with a long time ago. He was experiencing so much pressure to eat at the table every night, he simply shut down and wouldn't eat. While you might think his parents were threatening him to eat, it wasn't that way at all. He was asked several times during a meal to "take a bite," followed by "we know you'll like it!" Then, they moved on to lovingly requesting him to eat. "Please try it, Will." With no success, his parents would tout the health qualities of the meal, as if this would motivate him to try something new. Eventually, they couldn't help but show their disappointment and bewilderment at Will's general lack of eating.

Of course, Will's parents were worried about him and desperate to help him eat and gain weight. But their nightly pressure at the table created a cycle of early fullness, anxiety, and lack of interest in eating. Will continued to eat poorly and lose weight until his parents adopted a new approach.

Depending on your child's temperament, too much pressure to eat can work in the opposite direction and may lead to overeating, especially if your child desires to please you. In a nutshell, your child may eat more when asked, disregarding her fullness signs. Over time, when kids don't listen to their body's appetite cues, they may learn to overeat habitually. Certainly, both of these eating outcomes are the opposite of what many parents are trying to achieve. Yet, these are very real results and I see them in nearly every picky eating case with which I work.

If you have a new eater, consider this information about feeding styles and daily practices a "head's up." If you already have a picky eater, I'd like to you think about whether or not you're using pressure to motivate your child to eat and how pressure may be affecting your child. The following questions are meant to highlight any potential pressure you may be placing on your child to eat.

REFLECTION:

Is pressure getting in the way?

What do you (or your partner) do if your child says he's not hungry?

_____

_____

_____

_____

What do you (or your partner) do if your child only eats a small portion of food?

_____

_____

_____

_____

What do you (or your partner) do if your child does not eat everything you offer at mealtime?

_____

_____

_____

_____

What do you (or your partner) do if your child says he's finished eating and wants to leave the table?

_____

_____

_____

_____

THE SHORT-ORDER COOK

Becoming a short-order cook is also fairly common, particularly when you have a finicky eater on your hands. You may want your child to eat so desperately that you'll make her whatever she _will_ eat. It's a slippery slope and a trap that many parents of new and picky eaters fall into.

Donna was stuck in a cycle of making her daughter a separate meal every night. She didn't want to, and knew it wasn't helping the situation, but she didn't know what to do differently. "Giovanna just won't eat unless I make her chicken nuggets. She complains, whines, and generally makes our mealtime miserable unless those nuggets are on the table," said Donna. "And if I try something new, it becomes such a big ordeal."

Studies tell us that when parents short-order cook, or cater to their child's food preferences, children are less likely to branch out and try new foods.[27] They may even become pickier. Not only that, they may be more likely to suffer from nutrient deficiencies that can negatively impact their health and well-being.

USING FOOD AS A REWARD

Using food as a reward is another common practice described in the scientific literature. I see it used to motivate children to eat more, eat a certain food, or try a new food. Like the other practices mentioned, this too, may backfire.

Here's how food as reward plays out: You want your child to try a bite of broccoli, so you promise dessert if he does. The reward here is dessert. The target food or behavior is eating broccoli. You give the reward when your child performs the desired behavior. In this instance, when your child eats the broccoli, he gets the ice cream.

Studies that look at rewarding kids with food suggest that children's food preferences become altered, and not in a good way.[27] A child's view of the reward (in this case dessert) is enhanced, while their view of the target food (broccoli) suffers. A shift in food preferences and food hierarchy occurs. Bottom line: Using food, especially dessert, as a reward to motivate healthy food consumption or eating does not change food preferences for the better, or for healthier foods. It seems to enhance the preference for the reward food.[27] Furthermore, children are not likely to eat the target food (veggies) on their own when the reward is removed. In other words, a preference for the target food (broccoli) is not sustained.

If any of the feeding styles or practices I just reviewed sound familiar, it will be essential to change your approach to feeding your child. You'll need to drop the pressure, end the short-order cooking, and stop using food (especially desserts) to reward your child for eating. This will be critical in creating a positive environment that encourages your child to try new food. Don't worry, we'll dig into effective strategies in a bit. Keep reading!

STRESSFUL MEALS KILL THE MOTIVATION TO EAT

As you've learned, a feeding approach that is negative can cause additional stress for your child at the table. Stressful meals for any child are usually counterproductive. They may encourage resistance and emotional responsiveness in the child, adding to the stress for everyone. Stress may discourage your child from adding nutritious foods to her diet. At its worst, too much stress at the table can be the source of real anxiety problems.

Older children may experience additional stress outside of the home environment. The school-age child is strongly influenced by his or her peers, and typically wants to fall in line with what everyone else is doing. He doesn't want to stand out as being different. But if he brings the same food every day to school, or can't spend the night with a friend because there's nothing he can/will eat, or uses food modifications like pureed pouches, then he may feel different from his peers, left out, and perhaps even be bullied. All of this can cause even more stress.

Unwanted attention around eating may amplify unnecessary stress and anxiety in children who are selective with food. In fact, kids with extreme picky eating (ARFID) have been shown to have some form of anxiety, with 21% experiencing generalized anxiety and 58% having an anxiety disorder.[7] Often, in the older picky eater, it's the growing stress around eating with friends or outside of the home that prompts families to get more support and intervention. Two great resources about this topic are *Extreme Picky Eating* and *Extreme Picky Eating for Teens*, both by Katja Rowell and Jenny McGlothlin. A listing of other resources can be found in the Appendix.

Introducing new food to your child is not necessarily easy, nor does it have to be difficult. But additional stress, whether it is from your feeding style or practices, or outside influences, will always slow down the process. The goal is to make the mealtime environment as stress-free and positive as possible.

HOW TO USE A LOVE WITH LIMITS (DIPLOMATIC) APPROACH

There are three main areas you'll need to address to become more diplomatic in your feeding approach. They are: structure, boundaries, and reasonable choice. Let's run through the foundation of each and why they work so well together:

Structure really means having a routine schedule for meals and snacks. We covered the timing and components of these in Chapter Four. This regular routine becomes predictable for your child, while covering his appetite and nutritional needs. In other words, you know you're offering the nutrition he needs, at intervals that physiologically make sense. He knows he can rely on you to serve up food in a timely manner, which will most likely cover his appetite, provided he eats until he's satisfied.

Boundaries are the limits you set around food and eating. For instance, eating happens at meals and snack times; meals and snacks happen at the table; the kitchen is closed between meals and snacks; and no helping yourself to food without asking. These are all boundaries that help you stay in charge of food. They also help your child regulate her appetite and eating by upholding the structure (above) you've laid out.

Reasonable choice is essential to letting your child have a say without handing over too much control. Offer a reasonable choice that's limited to two food options. For example, you could offer your child peanut butter crackers or cheese and crackers for a snack. Let your child make the decision about which one to eat. When kids feel they are part of the decision-making process, they are more likely to be compliant, while building their autonomy. In other words, they have some 'skin in the game.'

You'll also want to practice Ellyn Satter's Division of Responsibility (DOR). Using her philosophy, you determine the details around the meal (what food will be served, when meals will happen, and where they will be served), and let your child decide if she will eat what you prepared, and how much. You can read more about this on her website, https://www.ellynsatterinstitute.org, and in my book, *Fearless Feeding: How to Raise Healthy Eaters from High Chair to High School*.

As mentioned earlier, using a Love with Limits feeding style, or diplomatic feeding style, is the most beneficial for your child. It helps him develop a healthy relationship with food, while promoting appetite and eating regulation, good nutrition, autonomy, and peaceful dynamics at the meal table.

While your feeding style and practices will always matter and influence your child's eating, the outcomes in this area don't wholly rest on your shoulders. Your child is an individual, progressing along a developmental spectrum with his own temperament. Let's look at how these two aspects may affect your child's approach to food.

THE INTERPLAY OF DEVELOPMENT AND TEMPERAMENT

Throughout childhood, kids are learning about their world around them, while governing their own bodies and behavior. Children are developing their own sense of self. No matter their age, they are moving along a continuum of development that is predictable and persistent. Food and eating are always part of this development, as children find their way with food, as well as other parts of their world. Understanding what's going on at each stage gives you valuable insight. In *Fearless Feeding: How to Raise Healthy Eaters from High Chair to High School*, you'll find a more in-depth review of childhood development for each age and stage as it relates to eating and learning about food.

For the sake of brevity, you already know that infancy is all about introducing new food to your baby and capitalizing on her receptive palate so she acquires new food preferences and a varied diet. Toddlerhood is the typical time for picky eating to start happening. It's also the time when feeding interactions between parent and child can get off track and negative feeding practices begin. In the school-age years, children are increasingly influenced by their peers, the media, and school. At this time, you may clash with your child about who's in charge of food in the home. The same goes for the teen years, though it can be more intense and you have less control. At all stages, it's important to allow your child to have as much say and control over their eating *as is reasonable*.

For example, it's reasonable to allow your child to refuse eating a new food, and it's reasonable to allow your child the ability to explore food without eating it (touching it, chewing and spitting it out, or playing with it). It's not reasonable, however, to think you can make your child eat, taste, or like new food. Those negative practices I described earlier such as cajoling, forcing, or punishing your child for not eating don't work in the long run. They potentially do more damage than good. It's also not reasonable to allow your child to dictate the menu for mealtime.

Getting into the mindset of your child also helps to understand your child's motivations and thoughts. This is especially important when you discuss food and nutrition. I've met parents who talk about food and nutrition in ways that would be difficult for another adult to comprehend. Remember, nutrition is an evolving science that is nuanced for each person. It can be confusing for adults to comprehend, so we need to consider the cognitive capacity of our children when presenting information about nutrition. The chart below gives you a sense of how children think and their developmental motivations:

The Toddler...	The Child...
Is a magical thinker	Is a black-and-white thinker
Is egocentric	Is a rule follower
Is self-centered	Loves to learn
Wants independence	Wants to belong
Wants control	Wants to please others
Has difficulty understanding basic nutrition concepts	Can think through a chain of events
	Begins to understand cause and effect
Cannot see long-term effects of eating choices	Lives in the present
	Makes rule-based choices

YOUR CHILD'S TEMPERAMENT

In each family, kids are different. I hear over and over about the family makeup and how one child is so different from the other. Even my own children will say, "We are all so different!" Honestly, that is a good thing, but it sure can make parenting harder! Particularly if you are trying to highlight and celebrate the differences in each child, rather than parent them the same way.

A child's temperament can be an independent force when it comes to eating. My own firstborn was a spirited child who wanted a say in everything. Yes, she wanted a personal consultation on every decision. When I finally recognized that having discussions, even if they didn't end the way she wanted them to, was incredibly important to her feeling heard—and resulted in better outcomes—my husband and I went with it.

You can witness your child's temperament around eating. Kids tend to fall into three groups:

The Eager Eater: Often parents call these kids "adventurous," and note they are willing to try anything. These kids accept new foods easily and accumulate a variety of foods in their diet quickly. They may also have a big appetite.

The Somewhere-in-between Eater: This category represents the vast majority of kids. They may be slow to warm up to a new food, but with repeated exposure and a positive atmosphere, they accept new foods over time.

The Cautious Eater: These kids are timid with new food. They need time to check it out, grow comfortable, and eventually add it to their food repertoire. Often, we see this eating style show up when solid foods begin. These children may be supertasters, have more sensory sensitivity, or be extremely picky.

Temperament isn't always so easy to determine by watching your child eat, however. While you may have a good understanding of your child's temperament, it doesn't necessarily translate to what you see in your child's eating. We can look to other aspects of temperament to give us clues:

Activity Level: What is your child's activity level? How much does he or she wiggle around when trying to sit still? Does he get up from the table frequently?

_____

_____

_____

_____

_____

Regularity: Is your child regular about eating times, bowel movements, and sleeping times? Or does she or he never seem hungry?

_____

_____

_____

_____

_____

Adaptability: Is your child quick or slow to adapt to changes in his or her schedule? Or do changes cause a meltdown or show of resistance?

_____

_____

_____

_____

Approach/Withdrawal: How does your child react to new people, new environments, or new foods? Does he or she engage and embrace, or shy away and avoid?

_____

_____

_____

_____

Physical Sensitivity: How aware is your child of noises, temperature of food or environment, changes in taste, or general "feel" of clothing?

_____

_____

_____

_____

Intensity of Reaction: How strong are your child's reactions? Is she energetic when laughing or crying or does she smile or fuss mildly?

_____

_____

_____

_____

Distractibility: Is your child easily distracted, or able to ignore distractions?

_____

_____

_____

_____

Positive or Negative Mood: How often does your child show joyful, pleasant behavior compared with fussy, unpleasant behavior?

_____

_____

_____

Persistence: How long does your child continue with one activity? Does she persist if it's difficult?

_____

_____

_____

_____

While the answers to these questions won't necessarily describe your child's exact temperament, they certainly can give more insight on the areas that may be challenging for your little one. Even as I wrote this part, I went down memory lane and realized my number two child was painfully shy around new people, experiences, and environments; yet when food was involved, she dove right in—the opposite of what you might expect.

What is most important here is to be aware of your child's tendencies and see if you can connect the dots with eating, so you can be empathetic. If your child has an intense temperament, this may show up in her eating. You may have a child who gets up and down at the table (can't sit still), digs in and rebels when you ask her to eat more, or who tosses a tantrum or two when disappointed about meals. Remember, you cannot change your child's temperament, but you can adapt your responses and your environment to help your child adapt better.

When it comes to feeding, you bring your feeding style and daily feeding practices to the table every day. Your child brings his temperament and developmental stage. Together, you navigate food and meals. This can be smooth sailing on some days, and a rocky road on others. Having a greater awareness of what you bring to the table will help you better navigate what your child brings to the table.

Your child's temperament and developmental stage will help form your approach. No matter what, you should always be patient and try to introduce new food with a positive, engaging, and relaxed attitude. Stay away from showing frustration, anger, or forcing food upon your child. That's the fastest way to failure!

Next, we'll look at your mindset when it comes to helping your child try new food. When you have a positive mindset, it will be easier to get started with your plan.

CHAPTER SIX

THE RIGHT MINDSET FOR SUCCESS
You achieve what you believe.

MINDSET IS EVERYTHING THESE DAYS. There are tons of resources on developing a positive mindset. Experts believe a simple shift in your mindset can change your outcomes. I believe your mindset is connected to your own feelings of success with nourishing your child, especially if you have a new or finicky eater.

In this chapter, I will delve into your food mindset, from how you label food to how you label your child, and how you can be the model your child needs to see. I then turn to your emotional reactions and your expectations. These little thoughts and attitudes about food and your child make a big difference in how you feed him.

YOUR FOOD MINDSET

I believe there's an optimal mindset that goes along with introducing new foods to children. It's a mindset of adventure, realistic expectations, fun, exploration, collaboration, and support. A positive mindset is not that hard to cultivate. Imagine the mindset you have when you're about ready to go on vacation. You're excited, full of anticipation, hopeful, and happy. Let's tap into some of that as we discover the ideal mindset for helping your child try new food.

Want to know what *won't* work? A mindset that tells you that your child will never like this, will never try, or will never overcome his pickiness. Negative, negative, negative. As many mindset experts will tell you: you get what you expect. In other words, if you believe it, you achieve it.

If you dread feeding your child because he is unpleasant, you'll find it hard to encourage exploration or adventure. And it will be hard to engage your child with fun experiences around food. If you call your child "picky" over and over, he may self-identify as such, and this prophecy will likely be fulfilled. If you give up with new food before you give yourself and your child some time to achieve some progress, you may end up blaming yourself, or worse, your child.

If you need to make some tweaks to your mindset, this chapter will help. Maybe it will be just what you need to stay inspired, hopeful, and helpful.

THE DREADED LABELS: GOOD FOOD, BAD FOOD & "PICKY"

As an extension of your mindset or the way you think about food, you may have some preconceived notions about food and about pickiness. Let's chat about this.

I am acutely aware of the sentiments about food in our world today. Partly because this is my "work world," and partly because I try to stay on top of what people are eating, thinking, and doing. If you're in the Bad Food Club, you probably think there is a lot of "junk" food out there. Maybe you refer to food as "toxic," "full of crap," or even "evil." I've heard all of these descriptors and more about food.

Personally, I refuse to categorize food as *bad*. As a pediatric nutritionist, I know how confusing the term "bad food" can be for a child. First, if your child likes ice cream, yet it's deemed "bad" by you, how will your child sort that one out? And what sort of feelings can arise from this?

I love ice cream. It tastes so good. But, mommy says it's bad for me. I must be bad because I like it.

Second, food is food. Yes, there is the good, the bad, and the ugly when we consider food. And, yes, you have full agency over which foods you choose to offer your child and stock in your home. If you remember Chapter Four, I placed sweets and treats in the Fun Food category so you could find a way to balance and include them in your child's diet. I don't demonize Fun Foods or tell you to eliminate them all together. Doing that would not serve your child. All food is legitimate. Demonizing certain foods is confusing and potentially damaging to the relationship your child is building with food, himself, and his body.

My best advice for you is to drop the "bad food" category and just refer to food as what it is: Food. You can certainly add descriptors, but let's keep them positive and educational, such as nourishing, energizing, Fun Food, a fruit, a vegetable, and/or a 'sometimes' food.

Equally as problematic is the glorification of food. Idealizing certain foods can set up a guilty complex, especially if you've got a child who can't quite bring himself to eat those "good" foods. Talk about guilty feelings!

I am very sensitive to the words that are used to describe food, particularly to children, and I think you should be, too. I believe they do better with learning, enjoying, and navigating food when you remain neutral about it.

Last, let's discuss the label, "picky." I know some of you detest that word. I know some of you relate to that word. I use the term "picky" in my work and interchange that with finicky, fussy, and selective. However, what I don't do is address a child with the label "picky eater." Labels can be detrimental and dangerous. Why? Because too many times a child will live up to that label. *Bully, bossy, sassy girl, picky eater*. These labels tell a child what she *is*, rather than describing her behavior. This is a subtle, but powerful difference. Rather than putting a label on your child, try describing the behavior *you want to see*.

When you embark on helping your child try new food, I'd like you to keep a few more mindset shifts in mind.

EMBRACE ADVENTURE AND EXPLORATION

"I wish my son was more adventurous with food," said Ann. "We can't go out to dinner because there is nothing for him to eat." The desire to have an adventurous eater is a strong one for many parents. It makes sense to me. Having an adventurous child means you can bring anything to the table for meal time. It means you can go to any restaurant to eat. It means you can travel the world. Of course, you want your child to eat everything, without hesitation or a fight. You want him to enjoy food, too.

Adventures are fun, unpredictable, and sometimes surprising. You can adopt this same spirit of adventure when it comes to trying new food, and I encourage you to do so. A sense of adventure comes from the parents and can be contagious. If you are oozing with an adventurous attitude, it may spill over to your child.

There's nothing more that screams adventure than getting your kids into the kitchen to cook. Research tells us over and over, hands-on learning experiences are the most fruitful, engaging, and transformative approaches for children. Yes, it's a mess. But, in the long run, it's totally worth the cleanup.

Have you watched little ones try a new food? It's fun to watch their unique personalities and temperaments shine through. Some kids are little analysts; smelling food, separating it, and touching every nook and cranny. Others are little scientists, mixing food with other things on their plate, dipping solids into liquids, or carefully separating food to make sure it doesn't touch another food.

Remember what you learned in Chapter Three about the sensory experience of food? Don't hold your child back from investigating food with all his senses. If you do, you may be robbing him of the opportunity to get comfortable with a new food using a different sense, such as smell or sight.

Also, don't forget your child was born curious, and this curiosity helps him learn about food. He will look for differences and be intrigued by the new and unexpected. Use this natural curiosity to your advantage.

No matter the tendency, every child has his or her own style of exploring food. My advice: respect it and allow it. The tactile investigation of food is part of development. It is necessary and productive. Eating and accepting new food is a learning process. Learning takes place on many levels, and at an individual pace. Don't be too quick to correct, distract, or stop your child when he is in exploration mode.

If your child is cautious and careful around new food, or fearful of new food, or if he shows complete disinterest, be sure to be extra patient and careful with your support. Continue to expose your child to different foods and eating experiences, but relax your expectations. Going too hard, too fast, or too intensely may be counterproductive and delay your child's progress.

BE A GOOD ROLE MODEL

The Walker kids were struggling with food. One child was demanding about his food preferences and was a big eater; the other child was choosy and barely eating enough. And manners? There weren't any.

Part of the challenge was the lack of family meals. The family infrequently gathered around the table together, as both parents worked late. Mom or Dad fed the kids earlier and would occasionally sit with them while they ate. (You can bet the pressure to eat was high!)

More often than not, the parents would eat after the kids were in bed. Mom and Dad preferred this because they followed a low carb diet and didn't want to be tempted to eat the kids' food.

When kids don't eat with their parents, they fail to get a daily injection of role modeling around the table. They don't get a model of balanced eating. They don't see an adult using manners and enjoying the food he eats. They don't engage in conversation, passing food, and waiting for a turn. Simply put: they don't have a role model.

Remember, kids aren't born knowing how to behave and engage at the meal table. They have to learn it. And they learn it from you, their parent.

As a parent, you are the most important and influential role model for your child. If things aren't going well at the table, you must step back and ask yourself, "Am I providing the model my child needs to see in order to behave the way I want him to?"

Rather than talk and tell your child what to do, show him.

> Kids aren't born knowing what to eat, how to behave at the table, or why they should choose one food over another. They need a guide and teacher. That guide and teacher is you.

BUILD AUTONOMY FOR GREATER SUCCESS

Many parents tell me they want their children to eat healthy on their own. In other words, they want their child to pick healthy options more often, without being told to do so. That's a lovely dream. But it's going to take some diligent work on your part, and some time.

What we are talking about is autonomy. Autonomy involves nurturing your child's capacity to self-regulate his eating when you are not around. It also encourages his personal ownership over food decisions and eating, including the behaviors and attitudes you are trying to instill.

Autonomy is the end goal. It means your child is able to make food decisions on her own, regulate eating using her internal appetite system, and manage her diet with or without you. Helping your child build autonomy throughout childhood involves several factors.

Nutrition education: How you teach your child about food and nutrition, including hands-on learning, guidance, and discussions.

Involvement: Whether or not you let your child be involved with food, including preparation and cooking.

Encouragement: Allowing your child to discover, taste, and explore food.

Praise: Sensitive and appropriate praise for food choices, eating habits, and other healthy lifestyle choices.

Reasoning: Being able to understand the intricacies about food and nutrition, which will largely depend on developmental stage and cognitive skills, and making decisions based on that knowledge.

Negotiation: Encouraging and hearing your child's "voice" when it comes to food preferences and appetite.

I want my kids to be autonomous with food and eating, and I bet you do too. How liberating to trust and know your child can navigate the outside world of food without telling her what to eat! That's the gold medal. The win. For you, and for your child.

If you have a new eater, autonomy is your end goal —the long-term vision. It's the same goal if you have a picky eater, it just may take more perseverance and patience on your part. And if you're dealing with the extremely choosy child (ARFID), you will have to muster more fortitude, empathy, and patience than you can imagine. Keep on trying and hang in there.

Look for ways to help your child achieve autonomy with eating and making food decisions, using the elements outlined above. Autonomy and independence don't happen overnight, but when you create opportunities for learning, allow natural consequences, and tap into teachable moments, your child will be on his way to successfully navigating nutrition in a very complicated food world.

YOUR EMOTIONAL REACTIONS AND EXPECTATIONS

When children don't do what we want them to do, it can stir up some emotions. They aren't always pretty. "I get so mad at my son when he won't eat," said Henry. "I just feel so frustrated and don't understand why he won't just try. I wouldn't get away with this when I was a kid … my Dad would *make* me eat!"

Frustration is a common emotion I hear from parents. Anger crops up, too. Even despair and hopelessness can appear, especially if you've had a fussy eater for a long time. You may feel that you are ineffective and have little influence or impact with helping your child get through this phase. Or you may be afraid of your child's reaction to new food, and want to avoid conflict. I can assure you, you do have influence, impact, and effectiveness in helping your child. In fact, *you are the key* to helping your child. Avoiding the situation or the negative emotions your child may display isn't helpful, either. Children need help navigating their fears and emotions, even if they involve food and eating.

If your own emotions are getting the better of you, you will be getting in your own way. Negative emotions are counterproductive to supporting your child. Your frustration, disappointment, and anger can be felt by your child. Maybe these emotions have motivated your child to eat in the past. It's okay to admit, "In the past, when I've gotten mad, my child eats!"

Here's what I know: When your child experiences your negative emotions, it can cause fear. Fear is a motivator for everyone. If your boss gets angry and erupts at you for messing up an important task, you will be very sure to do that task right the next time. Not because you have a desire to do the task correctly, but because you are afraid of your boss and his reaction.

Motivating your child with fear (whether intentional or not) is not productive. Whether you realize it or not, big, negative emotions from you can scare, intimidate, and immobilize your child. I'm talking about frustration, disappointment, anger, yelling, threatening, and out-ofproportion punishment for not eating. Fear-based motivation won't cultivate autonomy, a positive attitude about food and eating, or a life-long desire to explore and enjoy all kinds of food.

Your child is a work in progress with his own timetable. Sometimes, unexpectedly, a new food is a home run, while at other times, that food you thought would be an easy sale, isn't. If you're an outcomes-oriented parent, or an optimist, you might be expecting success every time you introduce a new food to your child. If you've experienced failure in the past, you may be betting on food rejection every time you introduce something new.

My best advice is to be truly curious about food and your child's learning, and leave your expectations about food acceptance or rejection at the door. Be hopeful and expectant your child *will* try new food, eventually.

We expect our children will learn how to read, ride a bike, and drive a car, given time and practice. To support them through the process, we are patient and positive. I encourage you to bring that same 'growth mindset' to the table and your child's learning curve for food. Your child *will* try new food and expand his food variety with practice, patience, and a positive environment. Expect he will overcome this.

REFLECTION:

Let's check in with the emotions that surface for you around your child's eating.

What typical emotions are coming up for you when your child refuses to try food or eat?

_____

_____

_____

_____

_____

Where do you think these emotions come from? (past childhood experiences, overwhelm, self-comparison to others, etc.)

_____

_____

_____

_____

_____

In what ways are your emotional responses helping or potentially harming your child?

_____

_____

_____

_____

_____

What positive emotional responses would you like to cultivate and foster?

_____

_____

_____

_____

_____

WHY FUN IS SO IMPORTANT

Food should be fun. That's the goal, anyway. Food that's considered "fun" shouldn't only be indulgent (candy, cookies or other treats). All food and eating can be fun, or at a minimum, a positive experience. When there's no fun or the experience is negative or stressful, food and eating can (and probably will) become problematic.

Not only will injecting some fun into the eating experience lighten the atmosphere, it will potentially capitalize on your child's curiosity. Here are some creative ideas to help you keep the fun in food:

Add Color. Make sure there is color on your child's plate. Fruits and vegetables add a lot of color, so be sure to include them in the meal, even if you're not sure your child will eat them. Color appeals to the eye and is associated with greater satisfaction with eating.[10] Additionally, colorful food is an easy sign that food is nutritious, or in other words, has high nutritional value.

Shape Interest. Cutting food into shapes such as squares, circles, triangles, and strips can peak interest in food. I'm not suggesting you turn into a "Pinterest Mom," designing every morsel your child eats into a Picasso-worthy piece of art. Who has time for that? I never ventured far from rectangles, four-by-four squares, and triangles myself, which was enough to keep my kids guessing and interested. That could be enough for your child, too. Sure, cookie cutters can make a plain square sandwich much more interesting, so if it's easy and you've got the time, go for it. If your child is young, be sure to cut food into bite-size shapes or finger foods that are easy to pick up and handle, which helps reduce the risk of choking.

Put It On a Stick. String foods like meat, cheese, fruit, and vegetables on toothpicks or skewers to make kabobs. Also, alternating cheese, meat, and bread, or fruit and cheese makes eating fun and interesting for a child. Transform a typical sandwich into a skewered sandwich. Be sure to supervise young children when they use sticks of any kind.

Build It and Your Child Will Come. Make a yogurt parfait by layering yogurt, cereal, and fruit. Stack waffles, peanut butter, and banana for a nutritious twist on the typical pancake breakfast. Build a cracker sandwich with meat, cheese, and spinach or nut butter, honey, and raisins. Or better yet, put the ingredients on a plate or platter and let your child build it on his own terms.

Use Taste Tests. When you're cooking in the kitchen, invite your child to come in and evaluate the flavors and texture of what you're making. Use a formal process including an evaluation form. Have your child mark the flavors he tastes such as sweet, sour, bitter, or spicy. Include an area for texture: smooth, crunchy, wet, or lumpy. And don't forget the overall rating! I've got a sample Taste Tester Evaluation Form in the Appendix. Most importantly, keep taste tests easy, low pressure, and fun. I'll talk more about this in Chapter Seven. Use small tasting spoons and tiny plates to keep it underwhelming and unintimidating. Remember, a taste test is a "taste," not a mandate for "eating."

Now that you've learned about mindset shifts and expectations and how they may influence your child's eating, I hope you have a better perspective on how to proceed with helping your child try new foods. Understanding your role, from your mindset to your emotions and expectations, forms the basis you need to begin the process of helping your child try new foods. Let's do this!

CHAPTER SEVEN

PAVE THE WAY FOR POSITIVE FOOD EXPERIENCES
"It's dinnertime!" yells Mom. "Yay!" says her child.

I F YOU'VE MADE IT THIS far in the book, you've learned a lot about yourself, your child, and introducing new food. You've learned the old advice is, well, old. Waiting it out may do more harm than good. You know by now that overcoming picky eating is more than putting out a pretty plate of food, or showing your child different shapes, sizes, and types of food. You know it's about taking action, but making sure that action is positive and productive. Getting kids to try new food is an art, requiring a delicate balance of the right attitude, positive feeding, good nutrition, and patience. By this point, I hope you've received that message.

As we move through the next chapters, our focus will be on practical techniques you can try. Some of these techniques should be your default approach because they are gold standard practices. Other tactics you may use by design. Based on your child and family dynamics, you may feel a particular technique could work really well for your child. Design your feeding approach to include those extra techniques.

Additionally, I will revisit the what, where, and when of new food introduction, and how to minimize distractions. I'll help you think about your next food "move" when deciding how to build upon your child's current diet as you move toward more variety. Along the way, you'll get tips for keeping your child calm and your mealtime stress free.

ON THE PLATE: FOOD DECISIONS

"My daughter has been so hard to feed for so long, I don't even know where to begin," expressed April. "If I'm honest, I feel beaten down, knowing there will be a battle or a sad child at my table if I venture off her normal food."

April expresses the fear and hopelessness many parents in this situation feel. However, I want you to remember, you're not a victim here. Your job is to help your child move along with eating food. You need to manage your emotions and let your child figure out how to manage hers. Even if you believe you have the pickiest child on the planet, you still have the same job: introducing new food and helping your child navigate healthy eating habits.

You're at a good place right now. You've already learned about food balance, food groups, and portions earlier in Chapter Four. Here, I'm going to build upon what you've learned and give you some practical guidance for meals and snacks. While you're aiming for a balanced plate that is colorful and full of nutrition, your child may not be ready for this yet. So how do you get there? I will help you!

First, I want to cover a few things about each food group, the concept of safe foods, and how you can keep food simple. Then, we'll discuss a process called *food chaining*, which will help you strategically choose new foods for your child to try.

SOME FOODS ARE HARDER TO EAT THAN OTHERS

When it comes to resisting and refusing food, certain foods rise to the top of the list. The biggies: protein, vegetables, fruit, and dairy. Grains, which are carbohydrates (or "carbs" as people call them), are typically well-liked and a staple in the picky eater diet.

Protein Foods

Protein foods, especially meat, can be difficult for kids to chew. Overcooked, tough meat is difficult for a young child or new eater to chew, and older kids may have given up or gotten lazy over time with meats that are simply not worth the effort. I have found that cooked ground beef or turkey, shredded rotisserie chicken, tender cuts of beef (e.g., filet mignon) or meat prepared in the slow cooker is flavorful, more tender, and easier for children to eat.

My One & Only Slow Cooker Meat Recipe, located in the Appendix, is my go-to slow cooker recipe for meats like beef and pork. It produces a tender meat that is easy to shred.

If your child is not eating a variety of protein foods, such as eggs, dairy, and meats, you'll want to keep an eye on iron intake and risk for iron deficiency anemia. Zinc and vitamin B_{12} are other nutrients that can suffer if protein foods are eliminated or not eaten very frequently. A multivitamin and mineral supplement in an age-appropriate dose can help close the gap. I've listed a few of my favorites in the Appendix.

Vegetables

Children commonly shun vegetables (for reasons I reviewed in Chapter Three), yet it's the one food category parents stress the most about. The good news is that you can offer fruit as a stand-in for veggies, as similar nutrients are represented in both. However, if you do this, *you still want to expose and offer your child vegetables*. That is the one and only path to helping your child overcome his dislike for veggies and help him increase his food variety in this area.

Adding fat in the form of olive oil or butter to veggies can bump up flavor and entice children to try them. A little bit of salt can improve flavor, as well. Using dips like hummus or Ranch dressing can make raw or blanched veggies come alive with flavor. If your child is a ketchup fanatic, it's okay to use ketchup as the common denominator for introducing different vegetables. Don't forget about other forms of veggies like veggie chips, oven-baked kale chips, edamame, and working vegetables into quick breads and smoothies.

If your child doesn't eat many vegetables or fruit, you'll want to think about using a multivitamin to cover important nutrients like vitamin A, vitamin C, potassium and more.

Dairy Foods

Some children don't like dairy foods, but I find this rare. Even if a child doesn't drink milk, she may eat yogurt or cheese. Dairy foods (and their non-dairy, fortified counter-parts) provide calcium and vitamin D (and other nutrients) your child needs for his developing bones.

Dairy foods also provide a source of protein, and if protein foods like meat are *not* present in the diet, dairy foods can offer needed protein for growth and development. Non-dairy milks such as almond, other nut milks, and rice milk are *not* a good substitute for the protein content found in cow's milk, soy milk, and pea protein-based milks. Nut milks and rice milk do not contain even one gram of protein.

If you want to learn more about calcium and how to make sure your child is getting enough, regardless of your dietary patterns, please check out my guide, *The Calcium Handbook* (available on my website, www.JillCastle.com).

Since you already know the ideal balance of food groups, use this knowledge to your advantage as you plan meals and snacks. Identify the nutrition gaps in your child's diet by monitoring and keeping track of his eating. For example, if your child shuns protein foods like meat, eggs, or poultry, or only eats one type of protein food, like chicken, this would be an obvious food group to work on. Similarly, if vegetables are missing or almost non-existent in your child's diet, you'll want to put some effort into bringing them to the table in creative ways. Of course, wherever there's a nutrition gap, you can fill it in the short term with a micronutrient supplement. However, your long-term goal is to move toward food acceptance and creating a varied diet.

A WORD ON SNEAKY RECIPES

"Aubrey doesn't know it, but I make her morning smoothie with kale and spinach. I sneak it in because otherwise I could never get her to eat any vegetables," said Kristin. Some parents, like Kristin, do this. And they do it a lot. They feel incorporating veggies into their child's accepted foods is the way to go. The *only* way to go. It's not surprising parents come to this conclusion. Celebrities and cookbook authors proclaim this is the best route to take. I disagree.

When I hear parents are "sneaking" vegetables into pasta sauce, smoothies, or muffins, a little part of me cringes on the inside. I don't have any inherent problem with putting vegetables in the blender, or boosting nutrients with "extras" in recipes and making food healthier. I'm the first person to encourage you to do that, as it's a creative way to make food more nutritious.

The problem is in *not telling* your child you've adulterated her food. What she thinks she's eating and what she is eating (in this case, drinking) are two different things. And when she finds out, it might not go down so nicely. In fact, that crucial trust and attachment we discussed in Chapter Five is undermined whenever you sneak or lie to your child about food. Between you and me, when Aubrey finds out her mom has been sneaking veggies into her morning smoothies, I think she may be less excited to drink them (and may refuse them).

Here's my request of you: Don't be sneaky with food. Don't try to sneak spinach into the morning smoothie, or carrots into your spaghetti sauce. Not only does this erode the trusting relationship you've developed with your child, you may find that hiding ingredients in the foods your child *already likes* may turn him off from them completely.[28] And what a shame that would be.

If you want to enrich your child's diet by adding nutritious items to his already liked foods, then *be transparent about it*. In other words, let him know you've done it and respect the fact that he may not want you to alter his food.

Learning and growing with food is just as much about trust as it is about nutrition. Don't damage the faith your child has in you as his feeder, as it will make the road to eating new foods longer and harder.

SHORT-ORDER COOKING AND 'SAFE' FOODS

One of the main goals for all children is to come to the meal table and feel comfortable and safe. One of my goals for you is to streamline meals and leave inefficiency and extra work behind. Choosy or timid eaters can be immediately turned off when they approach the table and don't see something they recognize and like as a part of the meal. For example, if you're serving a new dinner item, such as Asian stir fry with shrimp and vegetables, your child may be guarded, irritable, unwilling to eat, complaining, or asking for something different immediately. It's likely because she's not seeing something familiar that she likes on the table. In other words, something 'safe.'

Complaints, refusals, and drama can be quite a trigger, firing off anger, frustration, and inevitably, a search for an alternative meal. While your immediate instinct may be to make another meal for your child, or ward off the entire situation by cooking a different meal for her every night, that's not the answer.

As I briefly discussed in Chapter Five, short-order cooking is a negative feeding practice. Yet, short-order cooking is the dirty little secret of families dealing with picky eaters. Its sister, the "rescue" snack, is just as problematic. Remember, short-order cooking is resorting to a back-up meal (or an alternate dish) when your child refuses to eat what's on your table. The "rescue" snack shows up after dinner and before bedtime to assure your child doesn't go to bed hungry.

Let's play this out: You make a meal of spaghetti and meatballs. Your child refuses to eat it, and just wants pasta instead. You worry there is no protein in the meal. You ask your child what she would like to eat instead. She says, "Chicken nuggets." You make chicken nuggets. Let's acknowledge your frustration level here, and perhaps even some anger at yourself because you knew this would happen. You should've made the chicken nuggets ahead of time, right?

If you hold your ground and tell your child, "This is what we have for dinner tonight," but she doesn't eat, the guilt and worry gnaw at you relentlessly. When your child comes to you before bed and says "I'm *so* hungry!" you give in and rescue her with a snack. Sound familiar?

It's estimated that approximately 75% of parents give in to their child's food requests, or use short-order cooking, as a means to get their child to eat and relieve themselves of the guilt and worry that comes with a child who isn't eating.[22] In my humble experience, nearly *all* families have used some form of catering with their picky child. It's the path of least resistance. The peacekeeper. Yet, the irony is short-order cooking is largely ineffective. At a minimum, it slows down progress and makes your child less willing to try new food. *Why try something new when I know mom or dad will bail me out with pasta and chicken nuggets or a bedtime snack?*

Of course, there are short-term and long-term consequences of being a short-order cook:

- Your authority is undermined because you aren't calling the shots on food— your child is.

- You short change nutrition because you are serving the same foods and meals your child will eat. This maximizes repetition and minimizes variety, leading to nutrient gaps in the diet.

- While you've successfully placated your child, you may be left feeling frustrated and overworked, which can wear down your attitude, mindset, and ultimately, your demeanor with your child around the meal table. It's hard to stay positive about feeding your child when you're tired and frustrated.

- Picky eating doesn't get better, and it may get worse. One study suggests catering on a regular basis encourages picky eating, giving it life and *longevity*.

- The longer finicky eating lasts, the higher the risk of nutritional deficiencies, poor growth, anxiety around food, and social challenges.

There are a few things you can do to silence the short-order cook in you. For one, you can make sure to include a safe food or two at each meal. Safe foods are familiar and liked. They are foods your child has had experience with and can eat. This might be milk, fruit, cheese, or bread and butter. The presence of a safe food or two at the meal eases any anxiety by capitalizing on familiarity. Remember, familiar food calms, comforts, and boosts confidence for eating. *The goal: make sure there is something on your table you know your child is able to eat.*

Here are some tips to help you shed the short-order cook syndrome:

- Don't serve the same safe foods every night. Instead, rotate through the list of acceptable and liked foods your child has already acquired. (Remember, you created this list in Chapter Two.)

- Don't plan your family meals around the safe foods your choosy child likes. You only have to plan for one or two safe foods in the meal. Do, however, have an eye on which foods you'd like to help your child try, and plan ways to provide more experience with them.

- Close the kitchen after mealtime. Literally and figuratively. The kitchen is off limits and eating is over. This will encourage your child to eat at meals, rather than count on grazing or snacking later.

- Offer all the food groups at mealtime (protein, grains, fruit, vegetables, dairy, and healthy fats). The more food groups on the table, the more likely your child meets his nutritional needs and satisfies his appetite.

- Double up on nutritious foods your child likes. Got a fruit lover? Serve two types: banana and grapes. A carboholic? Do the same. Offer peas and pasta; or whole grain rolls and corn.

REFLECTION:

If you are short-order cooking, it is likely holding your child back from evolving into a healthy and adventurous eater. Answer the following questions as you begin to step away from this practice.

What situations lead you to short-order cook for your child?

_____

_____

_____

_____

_____

_____

What steps will you take to move away from short-order cooking?

_____

_____

_____

_____

_____

Which safe foods can you begin to add to your meals?

_____

_____

_____

_____

_____

_____

FAMILIAR FOOD BREEDS COMFORT

At the start of this section I mentioned that one of the main goals for all children is to come to the meal table and feel comfortable and safe. In addition to safe foods on the table as a means to increase comfort, your child will also benefit from a growing sense of familiarity with food. When a child sees something over and over, and becomes used to it, a budding sense of security unfolds. This comfort and security may desensitize your child to the offensiveness of certain foods, helping him grow more confident and willing to try it. If you think about your child's favorite foods, he sees them over and over, and this may be why he's hooked on them.

Familiarity breeds comfort. Experience with food and repeated exposure, whether it's a brand new, disliked, or liked food, are the cornerstones of helping children accept and expand their food repertoire.

We can capitalize on the idea of familiarity to further increase comfort with tasting a new food. If a new food has flavors or tastes your child has experienced before, she may be more willing to try it. For example, if your child had apple cake at grandma's house and liked it and now you are at a neighbor's house and apple cake is being served, you can say:

Remember you had apple cake at Grandma's house and you seemed to enjoy it.

This may or may not increase your child's comfort, but it provides a context and a memory for your child to think through as he makes his decision to try or not.

Alternatively, a novel or unfamiliar food with no frame of reference can make your child resistant to trying it. Whenever you can, connect the dots for your child and prepare him for a new food, using context or a reference point:

This [food] is crunchy like your favorite crackers.

I think this is what your best friend Luke likes to eat.

Daddy ordered this last time, and you seemed really curious about it…

You like pepperoni pizza and you like bacon. I wonder if we could put bacon on top of pizza?

We'll be having mashed potatoes at Aunt Jane's house tomorrow. I know you like Mommy's mashed potatoes. Want to do a taste test comparison with me?

SIMPLIFYING COMPLICATED FOOD

Kids prefer less complicated food over food they cannot identify or that may be foreign to them. My families tell me their child would never touch lasagna, goulash, or casseroles. I think complicated foods like this are intimidating to some children. Why? They can't see what's inside. They can't recognize the ingredients. Even if you tell your child what is included, it's likely not enough information to change their stance.

In my experience, keeping food simple and identifiable is the way to go. Part of this goes back to the sensory experience of food (Chapter Three). If there's a lot going on in a casserole or mixed dish—lots of color, textures, new smells—your child can get overwhelmed, feel out of sorts, and out of control. That's not to say that he won't eventually be able to eat casseroles and other amazing dishes, but for now, simplifying them can make meals a whole lot easier on everyone.

Deconstructing complicated dishes is one way to gently include these items in your meal plan. For example, separate the main components of lasagna into noodles, sauce, meat, and cheese, and let your child see them separately. Allow your child to choose the components to add to his plate. He may even build or assemble his own lasagna. Eventually, your child may be more open to trying lasagna in its whole form.

You can do this with other entrees, as well. Rather than put a pizza together or layer up a Fajita bowl, or compose the tacos, place the main components of the entrée in separate bowls on the table and let your child build their own. You've immediately shifted control to your child and probably minimized any drama, as well. Deconstructing complicated food is a good first step for children who are resistant to casseroles and multi-ingredient entrees. I have many examples of deconstructed entrees on my blog, The Nourished Child, under the search term, "Dinner Bar."

BRIDGING TO NEW FOODS (FOOD CHAINING)

Food chaining is a concept developed by the feeding therapists and authors of *Food Chaining: The Proven 6-Step Plan to Stop Picky Eating, Solve Feeding Problems and Expand Your Child's Diet*. Food chaining is a systematic method of identifying current and accepted foods in your child's diet and their characteristics (crunchy, sweet, moist, white). From this, you create a "chain," or link, to new foods. The foundation food is something your child already likes. The "chains" provide guidance for the selection of new foods to offer your child. Food chaining emphasizes the relationship between foods in regard to their characteristics, especially taste, temperature, and texture.

For example, if your child likes applesauce, then you might offer an apple muffin. Apple is the common link or "chain" to a new food. The idea is that if your child likes the flavor of apple, she may be able to try other foods with a similar flavor. Applesauce, apple cinnamon oatmeal, apple cereal bar, and so on. The flavor across foods is similar but the texture and other characteristics may be different. Herein lies the opportunity and challenge for your child.

You can create "chains" based on texture. If your child enjoys crunchy textures, you can explore crackers, crisp toast, or chips. This can lead to crunchy vegetables and crisp fruit.

If the temperature of food is something your child is particular about, you can explore new foods based on that criteria: Cold fruit, cold yogurt, cold milk, and chilled veggies; Hot soup, hot grilled sandwiches, and hot pasta. You get the idea.

You can also change and broaden the context in which your child eats an accepted food. For instance, if your child accepts plain avocado, you can add it on top of soup, in a sandwich as a spread instead of mayo, or even branch out and mash it into a basic guacamole, and eventually add the traditional spices like lime and salt.

And even if your child is hooked on less-than-healthy foods, you can still make steps toward expansion of his diet. One of my clients liked salty, spicy foods, so we made progress by using his love for pepperoni to spur taste trials of bacon, sausage, and spicy Sun Chips. While you may be thinking *this isn't the healthy food I want my child to eat*, please remember that every time your child tries and enjoys something new, his diet gets broader; but more importantly, his confidence in trying new food grows. For children who have fear or anxiety with trying new food, building confidence and overcoming negative emotions is key. I'll talk more about this in Chapter Eight. And for a more systematic approach to food trials, see Chapter Nine.

Food Chaining Ideas	
If your child likes....	**Then try this...**
Apple	Firm pear, such as Asian
French fries	Sweet potato fries
Chicken nuggets	A different brand
Chips	Veggie chips
Macaroni	A different shaped pasta
American cheese	Mild cheddar cheese
Raw carrots	Roasted carrots
Peach yogurt	Mango yogurt

Strategic food selection is important as you help your child try new food, especially if your child is very picky. It makes it easier for you and your child because food selection makes sense, rather than picking a random food you hope your child will try. It also allows you to think about nutritious food as your end goal. While a crunchy carrot may not be your first "chain," you can map out a path to get there. For those little ones moving through the normal stage of picky eating, you can still use the principles of food chaining to help you round out a balanced diet. At a minimum, you'll at least feel like your food choices are strategic and purposeful.

REFLECTION:

Creating food chains can help you decide about the next new food.

Which food characteristics does your child prefer? (crunchy, smooth, cold, spicy, bland, etc.)

_____

_____

_____

_____

_____

Based on these preferences, what "chains" to new food might be possible for your child?

_____

_____

_____

_____

_____

AT THE TABLE: TIMING, LOCATION & DISTRACTIONS

Parents ask me *when* they should introduce new foods. They also want to know *where* to offer new foods. And some have brought along all kinds of distractions that interfere with eating. The food environment is just as important as the foods you choose to offer your child. Let's explore some of the basics.

Timing Is Everything

Building on our earlier discussion about structure, feeding intervals of two-to-three hours for young children, and three-to-four hours for school-age children and three-to-five hours for teens promotes an appetite for eating. This will play to your advantage as you introduce new foods. Your goal: a hungry child at meals and snack times.

Some parents use the dinner meal as the time when new food appears. It's generally a new entrée or a new veggie that shows up at the table. Interestingly, many kids are not as hungry and are more tired at the dinner meal than any other meal, making this time of day not ideal for trying new food. Instead, find ways to try new food earlier in the day such as at breakfast, lunch, or snack time. You can still bring new foods to the table at dinner time using the safe food principle discussed earlier, but keep your expectations in check. A weary, grumpy child who has already eaten all day may not be open to new food at dinner. Also, don't do new food after your child has just had a snack (or has been snacking all afternoon), because she may not be hungry.

Toddlers eat frequently throughout the day, so bringing new food to meals and snacks is pretty easy. Make sure your child is rested and has an appetite. Don't do new foods just before naptime, as it's unlikely your child will have the patience and stamina to try it.

If you're lunching or snacking on food your child hasn't tried before, share a small piece with her. You can do this at dinner or when mealtime is winding down. Allow your tot to sit on your lap and explore your plate. Resist the urge to put pressure on her to try a bite! Let your toddler lead with her curiosity. Don't direct her.

For older kids, I advise you use after-school snack time as a time to explore new food. Children generally come home hungry and they're ready to eat. A snack platter can showcase a variety of food such as crackers, cheese, fruit, nuts, and fresh veggies for your child to explore. Because there is so much variety on the plate, you can slip in a new food, like edamame for example, and see what happens. At mealtime, use the principle of always having a safe food alongside a new food on the table, as described previously.

One tip that has worked for other families is to introduce a new food at the beginning of a meal. Grabbing five minutes before dinner to offer a small taste of a new food places the odds in favor of your child's appetite. If your child is emotionally reactive to new foods and this has ruined the meal in the past, you can try this pre-meal introduction technique and see if it helps. At a minimum, separating the introduction of new food from the meal may reduce pressure on your child and you may see your child be more willing to try.

If you're on a mission to expose and expand your child's diet, offer a new food once a day, or at least several times a week. You don't have to go to the store every week solely for the purpose of buying new foods to try. Rather, new foods can be the foods you enjoy eating, want to eat, and desire to have your family eat. If your child is eating chicken nuggets and you're eating chicken piccata, then chicken piccata is the new food. New food can naturally show up at meals and can reflect the family diet.

It goes without saying, but I'll say it anyway, if you've got a tired, sick, moody child and you sense the timing isn't right for new food, wait. A negative experience deepens the picky eating trenches. On the flip side, your child probably has more fortitude than you think. Use your parenting instinct to guide you!

Location, Location, Location

I'm a fan of having kids eat mostly at a designated table, island, or other location associated with eating. Even if you don't have a kitchen or dining room table, you can set up a coffee table or picnic blanket on the floor as your usual place for meals and snacks. This helps uphold that structure I described in Chapter Five and lets children know where eating typically happens. It also helps them focus on the food they are eating and pay attention to their appetite.

The reality is, however, food is offered *everywhere* and is fair game for trying. Your child will encounter food in his outside world—at school, daycare, church, play groups, relative's houses, restaurants, and more. When your child is outside his home environment, let him take the lead on trying new food. (If you're following my guidance in this book, you are already respecting your child in this area.)

Pressure to eat can be a real factor outside of your home and it can work in different ways. For one, peer pressure can be a positive influence on a toddler's or a preschooler's eating.[29] When young children in a social environment see others eating novel foods, they may also be inclined to try those foods; especially when the feeding environment is positive, pressure-free, and promotes autonomy.

I've seen many picky eaters blossom when they head to preschool. Being around other peer eaters, the explorative nature of preschool, and the multiple opportunities for autonomy with tasks of daily living, including eating, can inspire an openness to try new food in any young child.

On the other side of the coin, though, the outside world can serve up a different scenario. Pressure to eat from well-meaning adults such as teachers, caretakers, and grandparents is an all too common reality. Your child may feel the "heat" to eat.

"Try it, you'll like it!"

"Oh come on – be a big boy and taste it."

"Your mom was never this picky…where did you come from?!"

"We all take a bite to be polite in this classroom."

Although subtle, these comments and situations aren't helpful and can put your child on the defensive. At its worst, subtle pressure like this can cause a backslide to more resistance and pickiness. Be sure to prepare your child for outside eating events and guard him from situations that may be counterproductive to his eating. Don't be afraid to advocate for your child and address undue pressure with the offending adults in your child's life.

TV, iPads, Books & Games, Oh My!
Does your child need the television on to eat? Does she have a favorite program that gets played at meals? Do you have to make room for books, iPads, and toys at the table? Do you play games, sing, or incessantly talk to get your child to take a bite of food?

Is this your reality? My guess is you never thought you'd be here: singing, gaming, reading, and distracting your child in order to accomplish a simple task of survival. I bet you wonder how you got to this place of technology crutches and dramatic antics to get your child to eat. I know how you got there.

You've been sold on the 'distraction plan.' Worse, you've embraced the idea you have to get your child to eat, by any means possible. If you've come this far, I hope by now you know your job is to *provide food*, and your child's job is to *decide whether or not to eat it*.

The 'distraction plan' tells you that it's okay to divert your child's attention away from food and eating so you can slip in a bite here and there. It sells you on the notion that disconnection from the experience of eating is more valuable than connecting to the food you eat and your appetite. Worse, the 'distraction plan' disconnects your child from being aware and mindful of eating and her appetite.

Studies have shown that being present and mindful with eating creates more enjoyment while fine-tuning a sense of hunger and fullness during the experience.[30] Recognizing appetite cues (and acting on them) helps children eat for the right reason—hunger—and stop for the ideal reason—satisfaction or fullness.

Using distractions such as TV, online games, or toys to help your child eat promotes the opposite: disconnected or mindless eating. Distractions take the focus away from internal regulation of food consumption. Instead, it encourages eating for external reasons such as eating a number of bites or trying something new. The 'distraction plan' helps your child *tune out* of his appetite cues, rather than *tune in* to them.

REFLECTION:

What distractions are you using to help your child eat?

_____

_____

_____

_____

_____

_____

What approach will you take to wean off distractions at the table?

_____

_____

_____

_____

_____

_____

Distractions are a real crutch. You'll want to start weaning your child off them, gradually. If your child uses some form of distraction at every eating session, pick one session where you eliminate them. For example, if TV is always on during meals or snacks, choose one eating time like snack time when the TV is off. Gradually remove TV one meal at a time until you get to a point when the TV is never on during meals and snacks. Alternatively, define the duration of TV time by setting a timer. For example, set the timer for 10 minutes. When the timer goes off, the TV goes off. Gradually decrease the timer to 8 minutes, 6 minutes, 4 minutes, and so on, until there is no TV time at meals any more.

If you place multiple toys or books on the table during meals, place one fewer at each meal and gradually decrease the number until you get to one toy or one book at eating sessions. Proceed with dropping the remaining toy or book at each eating session, one at a time, removing them from another meal, and so on, until you get to none.

The goal is to have your child come to the table to eat. Not to watch TV and eat. Not to read and eat. Not to play games and eat. Removing distractions allows your child to focus on the experience of eating, including new foods, while building the muscle memory to internally regulate her own appetite. When we help our children focus on the task of eating, they will be better able to enjoy it, acquire mindful eating skills, and regulate their appetite and food intake.

The Ideal Table Environment

The table has to be a positive place for eating. Period. If there is a negative vibe, you (and your child) will have an uphill battle with eating and trying new food. Not only do you need a positive outlook, you need to thoughtfully create a pressure-free environment, a routine schedule, and the locale for eating. Refer back to Chapter Five if you need a reminder. Use your nutrition knowledge and food-chaining techniques to make strategic, nutritious food selections. Last, don't sneak, short-order cook, or distract your child to get him to eat.

If you can work on serving up a supportive table environment, your child is more likely to enjoy being at the table and this can lead to an easy, natural willingness to try new food. Creating positive experiences with food is so critical; many experts in the area of feeding and food introduction believe this can't be done successfully without ensuring the feeding environment is pressure-free and full of love, patience, and a nurturing spirit. I happen to be one of those experts. No doubt, adding new foods can be a long and tedious process (but it can be done!). And even if all this positivity around the table doesn't radically change your child's eating, know that in the long run, your child's memories of family meals will be positive ones.

In the next chapter, I will introduce some powerful tools to further help you guide your child in the exploration of new food. From family-style meals and a learning plate to ways to increase your child's food exposure, I've got more helpful techniques!

CHAPTER EIGHT

EMPOWERING TECHNIQUES TO ENGAGE FOOD EXPLORATION

Building healthy food preferences can begin with just one food.

W E DISCUSSED THE SENSORY EXPERIENCE involved with eating earlier in this workbook (Chapter Three). Besides tasting food, there are other ways to capitalize on food experiences, such as handling, preparing, and self-serving food. There are ways to warm up to food at the table, such as family-style meals and using a Learning Plate. I'm going to chat about these in this chapter so you have more tools and tips to draw upon as you move through this journey with your child. You may not need to use these, but you might. Especially if you've tried everything else.

The more experience your child has with food, the more comfortable and confident he may become with eating it. That's why using the natural laboratory of your kitchen can be very useful. I'll show you how.

In this chapter, I'll explore ways you can further allow your child some autonomy at mealtime and in the kitchen. At a minimum, you'll be teaching your child to have agency over his food experiences, something that will serve him for a lifetime.

"I've tried everything." I hear this statement a lot. Yet, when I run through my laundry list of techniques families can try, they usually haven't been tried. When parents say *I've tried it all,* they usually mean attempts at sneaking veggies, adding dips and sauces, buying different products, bribing with dessert, and waiting the whole picky eating thing out.

As you already know, waiting for picky eating to disappear or getting so action-oriented that you cause more problems doesn't work. I'm sharing some of the best, proven techniques to improve picky eating, or at least the dynamic around family mealtime. If you haven't tried these, you should.

If you're living with an extreme picky eater, trying these may help, but you may need more structure. For that, be sure to read the next chapter and learn about The Nourished Path™ to New Food, my systematic approach to helping picky eaters taste, eat and like new food. This can be used with any picky eater, though I tend to introduce this approach when families feel they are at the end of their options.

FAMILY-STYLE MEALS TO THE RESCUE

One way to expose your child to new food in a low pressure way is to serve family-style meals. If you're not familiar with this concept, let me take you back to a show that depicts family-style meals as the norm: *The Waltons*. It was a TV show about a family who lived in the Virginia mountains during World War II and the Great Depression. John-Boy, Jim-Bob, and Mary Ellen joined the family table every night with their parents, grandparents, and siblings. Platters and bowls of food were centered in the middle of the table. Food was passed around and each member served themselves.

This is the heart of family-style meals: Passing food, serving yourself, adding items to your plate, and deciding how much food to take. I like, use, and advise family-style meals for all families. I believe they are a game changer in helping children make daily food decisions, regulate their eating, and learn about all kinds of food.

Family-style meals have several benefits. First, they provide young children with opportunities to hone their gross and fine motor skills. Maintaining balance, passing platters, holding bowls, and scooping food are all motor skills that can be refined at the table. Second, kids can learn and practice their table manners. *May I please have, thank you*, *no thank you, my tummy is full now*, and other courtesies can be practiced and refined. Patience is naturally required, as your child waits for meal items to make their way around the table.

Family-style meals allow your child to choose which foods to eat from the items you're serving at mealtime. He also learns over time the amount of food that works for his body. Acknowledging your child's capability to serve himself and choose food promotes his growing independence and autonomy, not to mention the trust foundation we discussed in Chapter Five.

If you're working on diplomatic (Love with Limits) feeding, you'll be happy to learn that family-style meals honor Ellyn Satter's Division of Responsibility with Feeding. Not only do they allow your child to choose whether she will eat and how much, family-style meals respect the individual preferences and eating style of your child.

So, how do you *do* family-style meals?

After you decide what you're serving for dinner and prepare the items, place the meal components in the center of the table. Start the process of passing one item around to the person on your right or left. Pass items around in the same direction, one by one. Your child chooses what to add to his plate and the amount of food to add. Keep doing this until everything has made its way around to each individual at the table.

Generally, older children (over 5 years) can be independent with handling the platter or bowl of food and the serving utensils. Give support if needed. School-age kids are quick to pick up the routine.

Younger children (under 5) will likely need extra support from you. You can hold the platter or bowl and let your 3- or 4-year-old use the serving utensil to dole out a portion of each meal item onto his plate.

For even younger kids, allow them to tell you with their words (or signs) which foods to put on their plate or tray, and to tell you "when to stop" adding food.

For the choosy child who isn't trying new food willingly, family-style meals can expose your child to new foods in a natural and relaxed way. When food items are passed around the table, each child gets to hold, look at, and smell all the individual foods in the meal. Even if your picky eater snubs the broccoli, she still needs to be polite and pass it around, getting some sensory exposure in the meantime.

Another reason I'm a fan of family-style meals has to do with what they *don't* encourage. Family-style meals discourage parents from being "food platers." A "food plater" serves up their child's meal on a plate, selecting the food items and the amounts their child should eat. Often, this happens out of habit, without much thought for the potential long-term effects.

While some kids are easy going and okay with their parent being in charge of the meal selections, as you learned in Chapter Five, other kids may not be. This goes back to your child's temperament. For children, plating may feel controlling or restrictive. It may lead kids to react in ways that are counterproductive to their health (like overeating when they have opportunities for independent choice). If you pre-plate your child's food, you may also be inclined to overshoot portion sizes. When some kids see too much food on their plate, they're turned off or overwhelmed.

I bet you're thinking, *What if my child won't take any food? What if my child only takes what she likes?* These are common worries. If you go back to the principles of a balanced meal (Chapter Four) and the safe food concept (including one or two items on the menu you know your child can eat), you can allow your child to figure it out. Remember, success doesn't hinge on dinner. Be sure to offer nutritious foods throughout the day so that your child has every opportunity to meet his nutritional needs. Use a meal planning strategy that covers any food gaps along the way.

If you're serving new foods on the menu, encourage your child to take an itty-bitty amount on his plate, just for a taste. Don't use pressure, bribes, or threats. If positive encouragement stirs up any emotion, suggest your child put a small bite on a Learning Plate. Keep reading, I'll cover the Learning Plate next.

As you can see, family-style meals allow your child to take charge of his eating by choosing which foods to eat (from what you have decided to serve) and how much to serve himself. Many families I have worked with use dinner as a starting point for family-style meals because this is the meal that's the hardest on everyone. Ninety-nine percent of them tell me they see a dramatic difference in the calmness and mood at the table after starting family-style meal service. Remember, this positive, calm vibe at any mealtime is necessary for your fussy eater to open up to trying tastes of new food.

THE LEARNING PLATE FOR EXPLORATION

If you've got a child who won't willingly put anything new on his plate, then The Learning Plate is your next step. The Learning Plate is a small, separate plate on the table used for the sole purpose of food exploration. Learning Plates are good for any child who is hesitant, shy, or overwhelmed with new food. It can be especially useful for the child who does not want a new food, or experiences great emotion when a new food is placed on his eating plate.

The Learning Plate is helpful in taking the pressure off kids to eat new food. The purpose of the Learning Plate is to let your child experience a new food on his own terms and at his own pace. I tell kids who are using The Learning Plate that it's an easy way to train their taste buds with new food. A way they can warm up to new food in a gradual, low-pressure way. I remind them that sometimes we have to get used to new foods gradually, just like a new teacher, a new kid in the class, or a new sport. Over time, they can get used to the new food and be able to try it; and maybe even like it and eat it.

A Learning Plate is a tasting plate, not an eating plate. Your child can touch, smell, "kiss a food" (let it touch the lips), place food on his tongue and take it out, or even chew a bite of new food and spit it out politely in a napkin. The distinction is your child doesn't have to *eat* food on the Learning Plate, he can simply experience it.

The Learning Plate also allows you to tell your child, *"You don't have to eat it."* Some kids feel they have to eat everything when they come to the table. Even if there's been low pressure historically, some kids put the pressure on themselves to eat. *"You don't have to eat it, but this is a way you can try (or taste) it"* can melt away any pressure your child may feel about eating.

> Use this powerful phrase when starting with The Learning Plate:
> *"You don't have to eat it, but this is a
> way you can try (or taste) it."*

Not every child will need a Learning Plate, but I've found it's useful for kids who've experienced a lot of expectation and pressure at the table, either from well-meaning adults or from self-imposed pressure. It's also handy for texture and sensory sensitivities in the extremely picky eater, something I'll talk about in the next chapter.

There is a handy printable Learning Plate icon for you in the Appendix section of this book to help you understand and explain the Learning Plate to your child.

INCREASING FOOD EXPERIENCES IN THE KITCHEN

Getting your child in the kitchen inherently exposes your child to smells, sights, touch and more, kicking food exposure into high gear. Research shows when children are involved in making food, they are more likely to eat it.[31] Young children are particularly open to experiences with food in the kitchen. They love to stir, pour, peel, and crack eggs. It's one big exploration, which capitalizes on exactly what's going on with toddler and preschooler development. Older children like to be more involved in cooking and baking, which reflects their developmental drive to experiment. Find ways to bring your child into the kitchen, no matter his age. Select experiences that are age-appropriate and developmentally driven.

The Toddler Can...	The Child Can...
Touch, tear, stir, and sprinkle	Help with menu decisions
Learn about the color and aroma of food	Chop, cut, peel (with supervision)
Knead dough and mix ingredients with hands	Choose a new food to add to the shopping list (fruit, vegetable, or other)
Crack an egg	Knead, pour, slice, mix, assemble, measure, sift, and more! (supervise as necessary)
Peel fruit (banana, Clementine)	
Open a package	

Fun, Chores, and Big Requests

Getting your child in the kitchen to make muffins can be an overwhelming idea. Who has the time? The patience? With families on the go and busier than ever, the idea of cooking projects every day can send even the most well-intentioned parent running the other way.

You don't have to take on a big baking project every day. My guess is you probably don't have the time. I don't have the time for that, either. And, hey, it wouldn't work out so great for our waistlines and health if we did this every day, anyway.

But you prepare food for your family every day. Why not hand over some of that prep to your child? Have your child gather the ingredients for sandwich making. Hand over the knife and let your child spread the mayo or nut butter on her sandwich bread. Ask your child to put fruit in a bowl or slice some cucumbers and portion out little bowls of salad dressing for a dip. You don't have to do it all and it's not good for you to do so, anyway. When you think your child *can't do* something, I want you to figure out a way you can support your child so she *can do it*.

It's becoming more common for me to see kids who are hands off with food, rather than hands on. They don't use utensils to feed themselves. They don't open packages of food. They don't peel their own banana or Clementine, take the tops off strawberries, or cut their meat. While there are age-related limitations to some of these tasks, my point is that letting your child do for herself is an easy way to get her more involved with food and cultivate her autonomy.

While you may think your child cannot handle cutting his meat or pouring her milk, the truth is with a little bit of guidance, your child can learn. By becoming skilled in these simple daily tasks of living, she will gain self-esteem and a sense of capability, both of which are key social-emotional developmental milestones of childhood.

Chores around the kitchen also help your child's development. Taking out the trash, setting the table, loading the dishwasher or washing the dishes, and packaging up leftovers are just some suggestions for moving your child toward greater responsibility, more food exposure, and more involvement.

Of course, try to make all of this fun! Turn on the music, do a little dancing, or make a game out of kitchen chores to pass the time quickly and make it enjoyable. Try to be kind in your requests and clear with your expectations. Avoid arguments, threats, and punishments. Just as with eating, they don't work well to motivate the behaviors you want to see.

Taste Testers

Have you ever watched a cooking show? If you have, you'll notice that chefs taste their food a lot. They do this so they can evaluate the flavor of the food they are preparing and adjust the flavor components, if needed. They use small tasting spoons to get this job done. Often, you'll see a jar of spoons on their kitchen station or close by, ready for tasting anytime it's warranted or wanted.

You can use this simple concept in your own kitchen. Whether or not you set a jar of spoons on your cooking counter is not the point. The idea is to get your child involved in the process through small sample tastings while you cook and prepare food. Because this happens in the kitchen, the pressure associated with the dinner table can be avoided. Mimicking a cooking show doesn't hurt, either (small spoons, little dips, no pressure).

You can find small tasting spoons at party stores (plastic), cooking warehouses, and on Amazon. I have a colleague who created a small bowl and spoon set for the purpose of small tastes at the table or in the kitchen. Her company is called Brave Plate and her product is the Try Pod. It's simply a teensy-weensy spoon and a tiny little bowl. A clever way to separate the tasting experience from eating. Her contact information is in the Appendix.

You can make the tasting process more fun by adding in the element of a rating system. Your child can rate the flavor, smell, and texture of the food(s) he is tasting on a scoring sheet. I've got a Taste Tester evaluation form in the Appendix as an example. Adding this rating system makes this more of a tasting experiment, rather than another 'weird way Mom is trying to get me to take a bite of food.'

These kitchen-focused exercises increase your child's experience with food and keep the process fun. Creating chores, tastings, and hands-on experiences take the focus off mealtime and the table, while building your child's autonomy and experiences with food.

Of course, you won't have your young toddler chopping food or cooking over a stove independently, but several of these ideas can be started at a young age. As your child gets older and more mature, add in the more sophisticated elements. Beginning at a young age may mean your child gets more comfortable, autonomous, and adventurous around food (and perhaps avoids prolonged picky eating).

CHAPTER NINE

THE EXTREME PICKY EATER

When the timing is right, kids can gain confidence and courage with every food experience.

I F YOU'VE HAD A PICKY eater for a long time, this chapter is for you. The prevalence of extreme picky eating is growing and parents are looking for ways to deal with it (without making it worse). While the range of picky eating is quite wide, the extreme picky eater will always need the most patient, positive parent on the planet.

In this final chapter, you will learn about extreme picky eating, or ARFID, and the considerations and techniques you can employ to help your child, without harming the situation. You will be introduced to the structured approach I use in my practice with very choosy children who are stuck with eating. While this approach can be used with any child, I tend to reserve it for the more challenging picky eaters. You'll also read about when and where to turn for more help should your child need more support.

Eight-year-old Ben had been a picky eater his whole life. His family didn't know him any other way. In fact, they'd learned to live with Ben's idiosyncrasies around food. He would only eat one particular chicken finger from a summertime favorite restaurant, refused all vegetables, and preferred many sweets and snacks.

These tendencies weren't easy to live with and frankly, they sometimes caused quite a bit of drama in the family. Ben's parents had learned to skip the vegetables, not bother to offer other types of chicken, and live with meals that included cheese, crackers, and strawberries nearly every day.

Then Ben started to grow more anxious at social events with food and his peers. His growth started to slow down significantly. His parents started searching for more help. They learned Ben had an extreme form of picky eating called Avoidant Restrictive Food Intake Disorder, or ARFID.

Ben's parents had never heard of this term. They just thought they were dealing with a picky eater. But deep down they knew Ben wasn't your average picky eater. After all, he was eight years old and only ate a very short list of certain foods, prepared a particular way. He couldn't spend the night at a friend's house because there was nothing for him to eat. He was anxious, tearful, or argumentative at the meal table if his usual dinner wasn't there.

Picky eating had taken over, leaving Ben's parents to morph into short-order cooks, masters of bribery, and enforcers of more bites.

Whether you call this extreme picky eating or ARFID, it's a growing reality and category for children. ARFID is the diagnostic terminology used for medical billing and insurance coverage. It is a diagnosis given by a doctor or psychiatrist. Extreme picky eating is the common term used by many who live and interact with these youngsters.

For the purpose of this chapter, I'll use both terms. However, for ARFID, there are specific characteristics that have been outlined that need to be present for an official diagnosis.

THE CHARACTERISTICS OF ARFID

ARFID is characterized by a persistent disturbance in eating leading to weight loss or growth disturbances, nutrient deficiencies, dependence on liquid or multivitamin supplements, and impaired psychosocial functioning. The common signs are food refusal, poor eating or feeding skills, underweight or slowed growth, anxiety, and texture sensitivities.

If children are fearful of eating or are uncomfortable, why is this?

Kids with ARFID typically have an underlying reason for their food refusal.[7] In other words, there's a *why* behind their extreme pickiness. These reasons are many and varied. There can be a single persistent reason or a combination of reasons that keep picky eating alive in your child.

Early negative associations with eating such as a choking episode, frequent gagging, episodes of vomiting, or forcing a child to eat may cause a child to develop a negative association with eating.

Children with medical conditions may learn that eating is uncomfortable or painful. For example, conditions involving the gastrointestinal tract such as severe reflux (also known as GERD or gastro-esophageal reflux disease), or Eosinophilic Esophagitis (EoE), a chronic allergic response in the esophagus causing pain and inflammation, may place children at higher risk for ARFID. These kids may experience pain with eating and learn that eating hurts. Children with multiple food allergies are naturally limited by their food allergies and can become fearful of food and the possibility of an allergic response. A child with chronic constipation may learn that eating is uncomfortable or painful.

Sensitivity to texture or other food characteristics may significantly limit your child's eating or diet. Sensitivity to texture, smell, or sight can exist in any child. Kids with cognitive or learning challenges such as ADHD, autism, or developmental disabilities may also be at higher risk for developing ARFID. These kids often have sensitivities to food characteristics such as texture and smell. Sensory integration may underlie these sensitivities. If your child has problems with chewing or swallowing food, or neurological delays in development, he may learn that it's too tiring or hard to eat.

Children born prematurely may show heightened sensitivity in and around the mouth, particularly if ventilators, feeding tubes, or other oral manipulations were used early in life. Also, children who are frequently sick with upper respiratory infections and congestion may learn that it's too hard to eat when they're trying to breathe at the same time. Hence, they eat less.

Last, negative feeding dynamics may be layered on top of these root causes. Pressure to eat from parents, siblings, caretakers, and peers can further complicate any type of picky eating and stand in the way of progress. Pressure coupled with anxiety is particularly detrimental.

The reasons above aren't exhaustive. Each child I've worked with has had a different panel of reasons for their extreme picky eating. I've seen undiagnosed oral allergy syndrome (food allergy to raw fruits and vegetables causing itchy lips, mouth, and throat) and enlarged tonsils and adenoids as causes for extreme picky eating. Sensitivities to food characteristics (flavor, texture, appearance, odor) are a common cause, and frequently, ineffective food parenting goes along with many cases of ARFID.

Often, ARFID starts out as a child who is a fussy eater, a colicky baby, one with mild sensitivities to textures like clothing seams, or a child that never warmed up to veggies. The underlying reasons gain a stronghold, coupled by environmental influences such as parent feeding practices, other life stressors which may or may not cause anxiety, and recurring, negative reinforcement.

What sets kids with ARFID or extreme picky eating apart from other eating disorders is that they are generally not motivated to lose weight. Rather, they are motivated to stay away from the foods that cause discomfort, pain, or anxiety (stress).

If you feel you have an extreme picky eater in your home, there are certain red flags that indicate your child may need more help from a professional.

REFLECTION:

Check the signs of ARFID you see in your child.

- ☐ The list of acceptable foods your child will eat is short and shrinking.

- ☐ Your child eats food with similar characteristics (e.g., crunchy, same colored food such as all white foods).

- ☐ Your child has strong preferences for food preparation methods.

- ☐ Your child eats limited (if any) vegetables, protein sources (meat, beans, etc.), or fruit.

- ☐ Your child drops certain foods from his diet and never gains them back.

- ☐ Your child is growing poorly (or your child has a normal weight and growth, or may be gaining too much weight).

- ☐ Your child has signs of nutrient deficiencies (iron, vitamin A, and vitamin C are most common).

- ☐ Your child avoids one or more food groups.

- ☐ Your child is emotional or anxious around unfamiliar foods.

- ☐ Your child's social life is limited by his eating habits and food limitations.

My advice: If your child's picky eating isn't getting better by the end of the fourth year, it's time to look deeper and consider professional intervention.[6] As your child is entering school (e.g., kindergarten or pre-school), you should be seeing your child *add* foods to his diet, become more interested and willing to try new food, and gain better self-control of her emotions (e.g., fewer emotional outbursts related to food) in food-centric situations.

In my experience, the extreme picky eater rarely finds resolution on his or her own. When the extreme picky eater gets outside help, whether from a treatment team, a feeding therapist, a dietitian/nutritionist like me, and/or a counselor, she can make progress and experience success with eating, and even say goodbye to picky eating, eventually.

TREATMENT OF ARFID

ARFID and its treatment and management is still in its infancy. Research is afoot and we are learning what is effective and beneficial. Each child will be different in his reasons for ARFID, and therefore, the approach to treat it must be individualized. Help for ARFID generally includes food exposure therapy, learning about positive food parenting, boosting growth and nutritional status, and managing stressors related to eating. For example, children with sensitivities to the sensory components of food will likely need food desensitization and exposure-based food therapy with a feeding specialist. Kids who are anxiety prone will need help with coping skills, food exposure therapy, and building confidence around new food, and eating in social situations. Children who have experienced pressure to eat, bribery, or even punishment for not eating will benefit from parent-centered, positive feeding education, as well as other treatment approaches. Children who are nutritionally compromised will need nutrition therapy to restore nutritional health and improve growth.

Fortunately, there are teams who can treat children with ARFID, as well as single providers who can help. I've listed some resources in the Appendix. ARFID treatment can be achieved in a treatment facility setting, in individual counseling sessions with a feeding therapist, registered dietitian, and/or psychosocial therapist/counselor, or another treatment avenue. At the time of this writing, children with ARFID are receiving help in a variety of settings, from eating disorder treatment centers and hospitals to local private practitioners who specialize in this area. ARFID looks different for every child, so do your research to see which treatment setting is the right one for your child. The goal for any child with extreme picky eating or ARFID is to normalize eating, improve nutritional status and growth, and reduce anxiety around food so that your child can thrive in his life.

THE ROLE OF ANXIETY

Kelsey was a terrific student. She had lots of friends at school. She was an advanced soccer player and the youngest girl on her travel team. In every area of her life she was a shining star. But there was a troubled side to Kelsey.

Her mom described, "Kelsey is extremely picky. In every other area of her life, she's doing great. But when it comes to eating, she's rigid, resistant, and argumentative. We don't get it. We just want to help her get a handle on this part of her life. We see her struggle. And it's getting worse. I fear she is losing friends because she can't go to sleepovers or parties. If she does go, there's this whole production around food. I have to call the friend's mom and see if there will be something she can eat. Often, she goes and I have to send food with her. Lately, she's saying she doesn't want to go."

Nutritionally, Kelsey was a "white food" girl, eating pasta, chicken, crackers, milk, and cheese. No fruit. No veggies. No whole grains. There was more missing from her diet than present in her diet. When I met her, she was slight in appearance. It was hard to believe she was such a good soccer player by looking at her. She was sallow and had thin, stringy hair. She was polite but very quiet, avoided eye contact with me, and looked at her mom for answers and approval.

While I'm neither a therapist nor a specialist in anxiety, I can often recognize anxiety when I see it. It doesn't always look like the fidgety, nail-biting, foot swinging image we are told to expect; although it certainly can look like that. I suspected early on that Kelsey was not only dealing with extreme picky eating, but anxiety as well.

In kids with ARFID, or extreme picky eating, anxiety has been shown to be an underlying component, and a real barrier to recovery if left unaddressed. Some with ARFID have anxiety, and some may have an anxiety disorder.[7]

Signs of Anxiety in Children

Restlessness	Refusing to go to appointments
Agitation	Meltdowns about food on the plate or food touching
Inattention, poor focus	
Stomachache	Meltdowns about not getting preferred foods
Headache	
Avoidance	Hair pulling
Crying, temper tantrums	Eyebrow, eyelash pulling
Refusing to eat	Difficulty going to bed, sleeping
Refusing to come to the table	Type-A performer (in schoolwork, sports, etc.)

Anxiety can take on a life of its own. Little, random behaviors which may be categorized as *off, odd, or weird*, can become more consistent and persistent. In Kelsey's case, her mom noticed she started to wash her hands more, refused to touch food, and soothed herself by pulling on her hair.

Accelerating behaviors which are becoming more prevalent in your child's life may signal that your child is developing rituals, which may be a sign of obsessive-compulsive disorder (OCD). Obsessive-compulsive behavior may develop as a way to cope with strong feelings of anxiety. These are negative coping skills for feelings your child is having difficulty managing.

In my experience with extreme picky eaters, nearly every child has had some degree of anxiety. I've seen mild and more extreme scenarios. These kids benefit from therapy to help them develop effective coping skills so that their anxiety can be minimized. Think about it: It's hard to be brave and try new foods when you experience a significant amount of stress at the table, whether it stems from the food itself or from the family dynamic at mealtime, or both. If you sense your family dynamic around feeding is having a negative impact on your child, re-read Chapter Five.

In the older child, social situations where food is present may become a source of angst, as in the case of Kelsey. Often, social limitations are the trigger for families wanting to get more help for their child. What your family has been able to deal with in the home becomes unmanageable for your child in her social life. Equally challenging is the shame and embarrassment your child may feel about her diet and eating habits around her friends.

If your child is anxious around food or could benefit from positive coping skills, don't be afraid to get help from a psychologist trained in childhood anxiety. Cognitive behavioral therapy is a common approach, but I've heard of other approaches having benefit as well. On my podcast, The Nourished Child, I interviewed the author of *Sad, Perfect*, a novel about a girl with ARFID, and how she overcame it. This episode (#58) may give you comfort if you have a child with ARFID.

As I told Kelsey's family and my other clients, anxiety is a barrier to overcoming extreme picky eating. Anxiety will get in the way of progress and recovery. It needs to be addressed sensitively and effectively by a trained professional. And as an added benefit, helping your child develop positive coping skills will last a lifetime.

INTRODUCING NEW FOOD WITH EXTREME PICKY EATERS

Throughout this book, you've learned about the food needs, feeding interactions, mindset, and patience required to effectively introduce new foods to new and picky eaters. You will need all those skills to help the child with extreme picky eating, times ten. The extreme picky eater will need more support, patience, and leadership from you.

For example, children who are extremely picky (ARFID) may need more positive experiences with food than the research highlights. Some experts working with ARFID state that those children may need over 50 food exposures before they warm up and accept new food into their diet. That requires a lot of positive feeding interactions and patience from any caretaker. And some children, just like some adults, may never grow to like a particular food, even with intensive work. That's okay. We have thousands of foods available in our world. Your child *will* be able to accumulate an array of new foods into his diet in time.

However, with the extreme picky eater, you will need to take a more structured approach. This won't necessarily expedite the process (my experience tells me progress is slow), but it will keep things positive and moving forward, even if it is slow. In my work with extreme picky eaters, I take a few extra steps to set up a structured approach to trying new foods. It involves daily food tastes of food your child chooses with guidance from a caretaker or professional, evaluation of the experience, and tracking of progress. Following are the basic principles I use to help children move forward with food. You'll want to add these techniques to all the information you've gathered thus far in this workbook, especially the positive, sensitive approach to guiding your child through this challenge. If at any point, this process is worsening your child's behavior or anxiety around food, take a break. It goes without saying— but I'll say it, anyway—your child needs to be on board with this structured process. He needs to be motivated and want to participate.

THE NOURISHED PATH™ TO NEW FOODS (MY SYSTEM)

I developed this system when I worked in my private practice in Nashville. I developed it out of necessity. I had my first ARFID case back when there was no official diagnosis of ARFID. My patient was an 8-year-old, extremely picky eater whose eating, anxiety, and social dysfunction was negatively influencing the family dynamic. He was an active, overweight, sports-loving boy with lots of friends; but a very limited diet and a lot of angst around family mealtime.

Over the years, I have tweaked this system and use it in my work today. I use a lot of intuition in applying this approach to my clients. It's not for every child or every family. In fact, it's easier for me to tell you *who* it *won't* work well for: The child with autism, severe ADHD, or other developmental delay or neurological condition; and/or the child with significant anxiety around food and eating (this needs to be addressed first). These kids will probably do better with a treatment program supported by an extensive treatment team. Families who do well with my system are motivated to do the daily and weekly work. They are consistent with the program and persistent. They embrace food trials as much as they do positive food parenting and patience. This combination and attitude is the secret to success with my system.

If you choose to experiment with my program, you'll be setting up a weekly "Try-It Bite" system that promotes trying three small bites of different foods daily. Work together with your child (letting him be part of the food decisions and process) to make this a pleasant experience. Your child can help brainstorm foods he wants to try, can offer input about where to do food trials, and be involved or independent with tracking progress. For some families, getting a professional involved in this step is useful, especially if there is a history of distrust and negative feeding.

If you have a young toddler, you can select food options yourself, based on food chaining principles and other knowledge of your child.

Choose Try-It Bite Foods for the Week

Each day, your child will try three small bites of food. These foods will change weekly. Work with your child to select foods that he has an interest in trying. This can be something he's tried in the past, a food his friends eat that has piqued his interest, or a suggestion made by you based on the food-chaining principles we reviewed in Chapter Seven. Use the Try-It Bite form in the Appendix to outline your child's foods for the week.

Start all Try-It Bite tastings with a crunchy food, like a plain saltine cracker, to prime the tongue and mouth for new textures and flavors. Have a glass of water on hand for clearing the palate between tastes.

Tastings: Privacy, Please

Some kids are highly sensitive to the environment in which they are trying new foods, especially if they are experiencing or sensing pressure from family members. I ask my little clients where they'd like to do their tastings. I emphasize that all food tastings occur in a setting that is stress- and pressure-free. This is often in a private area. Sometimes it's in the dining room, a parent's office, or a nook. It's not at the dinner table at dinner time, or the snack counter with siblings, unless your child has expressly asked for that (and some kids will ask for that).

If the child is old enough, he or she can try new foods alone. If it's a younger child, trying a new food with a trusted adult works too. The main goal is to make this a pleasant, pressure-free, private environment. No demands to speed things up!

Less Is More: Small Bites and Few Foods

Keep in mind that large servings of food can be overwhelming. Insisting on big bites has the same effect, potentially shutting down appetite and turning off a desire to try new food. The goal is to *underwhelm* your child with food tastings. Use the size of your thumbnail or pinky nail to gauge the size of a bite or taste.

Additionally, don't make your child try five new foods at a time. Keep it to two or three foods… or even one new food. Work with these selected foods for a week, then pick two to three new foods for the following week (with your child's input).

Tasting or Testing?

For some children with ARFID, you'll have to begin with touching, smelling, and interacting with food. For example, I've had children peel a hard-boiled egg or a Clementine. I've asked them to cut food, or open a package of food, or simply smell different spices. Touching a new food or holding it counts as progress for some extreme picky eaters. You may need to establish this tolerance level before progressing to an actual taste of food. Your child may need to take the path of small milestones before actually putting food in his mouth.

How to Track Success and Setbacks

On the Try-It Bite Evaluation form, there is space to track your child's impression of the food he has tasted. I use an up arrow, down arrow, and sideways arrow to have children express their feelings and experience with a new food.

An up arrow means your child liked the food he tasted. You can add this food to your child's master list of liked foods (found in the Appendix) and work it into daily meals and snacks. A down arrow means he disliked it. Praise your child for trying it. Let him know you'll finish out the week with this try-it bite food trial because it can take several tries to warm up to a new food. If after a week of trying your child is still giving the food a down arrow, then table that food for repeat trials in the distant future. There are lots of new foods to try! Any and all foods can make a reappearance for a food trial in the future, so don't get hung up on broccoli as something your child *has* to conquer.

A sideways arrow means he's not sure whether he likes or dislikes a new food. Your child can decide to keep working on this food the following week, or schedule it for a future week to try again. On the evaluation form, there is also a space to write down the *why* behind your child's experience. Why did he like the food? Was it sweet, crunchy, or spicy? Encourage your child to write it down (or do it for him).

Equally as important, you'll want to know why your child didn't like a food. Was it slippery, mushy, or bitter? Write it down. This is important information that will guide future new food suggestions, and highlight areas that need more work, such as certain textures or flavors.

Respect and Praise

Always offer respectful praise to your child for his efforts, and acknowledge that trying new food isn't easy. Don't go overboard, though. Too much praise can be counter-productive to moving forward. In fact, I prefer parents take a business attitude to the whole process. Like strapping the seatbelt when your child gets into the car or brushing his teeth before bed, Try-It Bites are part of the daily process. The less attention and drama around the process, the better.

Your child may have days he's not motivated to do his Try-It Bites. Help him through this. Remind him of the little time it takes to do the Try-It Bites (less than 5 minutes), of his progress, and of his goals. Your child may have the goal of eating pizza at his sports banquet, or spending the night at a friend's house. Naming a goal can be motivating for your child.

There will be times when it doesn't make sense to do them, especially when your child is sick or your family is traveling. Do your best to stay as consistent as possible, and if you get off track, get back on the program as quickly as you can. When you do so, your child will make progress.

Tracking Progress

Many children are visually motivated. They like to see charts and graphs. If your child is a kid who likes concrete feedback, tracking his progress can be very empowering. Of course, if this isn't a motivator, or is contributing to anxiety or OCD, don't track progress with your child. You can, however, do it for yourself; and I encourage you to do so. Not every child will respond to tracking progress, so use your best judgment about including progress charts for your child. I find it works best to use them after your child has been working on trying new foods for a couple of weeks. But again, it depends on your child.

Keep a running list of new foods that have been accepted or added to your child's diet (check the Appendix). Letting your child watch his progress and growth over time can be rewarding and motivating. Additionally, it can build confidence to try other new foods.

You can also use this master list of liked foods when packing lunches for school. One thing I hear from parents is that lunches are the same every day and there's no variety in them. Once you have a master list, however, your child can use it to choose different foods for lunch. You can create a template for lunch choices. Highlight and group liked foods into a list that can be circled and selected for a packed school lunch. For example, if your child has three types of entrees he'll eat for lunch, three fruits, and four different snack items, then he can select a different lunch combination from the liked foods on his master list. This helps you know what to pack and lets your child have a say in the matter.

AVOID MISTAKES THAT PREVENT PROGRESS

It's easy and common to make mistakes while introducing new food to kids, especially with extreme pickiness. This workbook is an attempt to help you understand your child better and prevent mistakes. You already know that putting on the pressure or fighting with your child at the table are counterproductive actions. Yet, in the child with extreme picky eating, the frustration level can run high. Mom and Dad can see things differently and use different feeding approaches, making mealtime a hotbed of emotions for their child.

Children with ARFID seem to be more sensitized to their parents' emotions and may be more negatively affected by them. I can't emphasize enough that high anxiety and high emotions from anyone will almost always hold your child back from making progress.

If you're struggling, go back and re-read Chapters Five and Six. If you are thoughtful and deliberate, however, you can avoid these mistakes and the fallout that can happen. Do your best to support your child through role modeling, a calm demeanor, and an empathetic approach.

REFLECTION:

Which feeding mistakes keep coming up for you?

_____

_____

_____

_____

_____

Are there any nutrition mistakes you need to focus on changing?

_____

_____

_____

_____

FORCING, THREATENING, AND PUNISHING

Dramatic title, I know. Forcing a child to eat is not something parents like to talk about or admit. If you are following that little mouth left and right with a spoon full of food, or squeezing those chubby cheeks to slip food into your child's mouth, or making your child sit at the table until he eats a certain amount, you are forcing your child to eat.

In my mind, forcing boils down to using your authority or physical size to overpower your child with your will. Forcing almost always causes problematic eating because your child has no control over the situation. As kids get older, parents who may have used force learn that it doesn't work. A more subtle form of forcing, however, is making your child sit at the table until he does eat; or threatening to punish him if he doesn't eat by removing privileges like TV time, dessert, or other valued items.

Motivating a child to eat by using threats of punishment doesn't work, either. In fact, it can be damaging. Research has suggested that children who were forced to eat experienced strong conflict that resulted in crying, nausea, and vomiting.[32,33] They also experienced negative emotions and feelings including anger, fear, disgust, humiliation, and confusion. Furthermore, the foods that kids were forced to eat became the foods they _avoided_ later in life.

Remember Meg from Chapter Five? She wasn't allowed to leave the table until she finished her green beans, sitting many nights until late in the evening. To this day, she still can't bring herself to eat green beans.

Forcing, threats, and punishment don't work. In fact, they backfire.

KEEP THE FAITH

If you're a parent, the odds are you will face a picky eater. Whether you have a toddler or a pre-teen, a new eater or an extremely picky eater, this workbook was designed to give you some tried and true strategies for introducing new foods to your child.

The good news is there are small changes you can make to help your child. From changing the foods you offer to changing your mindset and feeding approach, there are many tweaks you can make. I hope this workbook helps you sort through the areas of change that make the most sense for you and your child.

What I want most for you, though, is to keep the faith. Don't lose hope. Don't fall prey to frustration and give up. Most children who are picky eaters are going through a developmental phase. They usually overcome it, especially when they get the parent support they need. You met Isabella in Chapter One. She was an example of a typical picky eater. With time, patience from her parents, regular new food introduction, and a feeding strategy that was predictable, she managed to work through this phase.

Isabella's parents didn't need to *make* her get through the picky eating phase. They didn't give in to her food preferences; rather, they offered a familiar food at meals alongside a new food. They didn't yell, force, or punish her when she didn't eat, but they adhered to their schedule and allowed her to get hungry if she chose not to eat or didn't eat enough. They didn't plan meals around what she would eat; rather, they selected meals based on what *they* wanted to eat, adding her safe foods to the menu. Isabella's parents trusted themselves (and their child) and the strategy they had in place for feeding her and exposing her to new food. They let Isabella work within *their* parameters, having faith she'd figure it out. Their approach worked.

You met Graham in Chapter One and Kelsey in this chapter. As extremely picky eaters, each of them has made tremendous progress. Graham overcame extreme picky eating with extra help. He used the Try-It Bite program of regular food exposure at home and in my office. His parents revamped their feeding structure, mealtime dynamic, and feeding approach at home. Graham's anxiety was addressed in counseling. Over a year or so, Graham moved from a stubborn, resistant eater who was melting down at the dinner table and only eating a limited list of foods, to one who embraced new, exotic dishes and proudly enjoyed his triumph over his past food fears.

His mom told me, "Last night Graham proceeded to make himself a plate of chicken, pasta with sauce, romaine lettuce with balsamic vinegar, and some fruit. He looked at his plate, and everyone else's, and said, 'Look how good my plate looks tonight!'"

Kelsey is a work in progress and continues to make strides. She has been through food exposure therapy, building a master list of 25+ new foods that she enjoys eating. She gained weight and replenished her nutritional status with a combination of new, nutritious foods, and multivitamin and mineral supplementation. During our work together, Kelsey continued to deal with anxiety, particularly around performance. Eating, sports, and academic performance seemed to trigger and exacerbate her anxiety. She is currently taking a break from food exposure therapy and working on coping skills to address her anxiety.

As you can see, overcoming extreme picky eating often requires additional help. Help can be focused on your child, or focused on supporting you and your parenting. How do you know you need extra help? If you are hitting the wall of frustration and feel that you are in over your head, if you've run out of ideas (or steam), or you recognize that things have gone too far and your child is getting worse, not better, then you should seek extra help.

MY BEST WISHES

I wrote this workbook to help you move from theory to positive action. Many parents tell me that they know they're supposed to offer new food without pressure. They are familiar with the Division of Responsibility and understand the concepts. They know they aren't supposed to be a short-order cook. Yet, what they don't know is *how* to take these "Do's and Don'ts" and turn them into an effective, practical, achievable plan for their child. So, consider this your guide to go from theory to practice.

If you've done the work here, you're on your way to using nutritious food, positive feeding, and effective strategies to introduce new foods to your child. You've begun the process of changing the things that aren't working for your child and incorporating new strategies you may not have tried yet. By the time you've arrived here, I hope you have a new strategy for helping your child broaden his diet, lose the fear of trying new food, and shaping yourself into a more effective food parent.

This *Try New Food* workbook can help any eater taste, eat, and like new food! Don't keep this workbook a secret. Share it with other parents you know who are facing challenges with introducing new foods to their children.

APPENDIX

APPENDIX A:

GROWTH CHART RESOURCES

Growth: Baby & Child Growth Charts by Clafou Ltd
https://itunes.apple.com/us/app/growth-baby-child-charts/id446639811?mt=8

Pediatric Growth Charts by Boston Children's Hospital
https://itunes.apple.com/us/app/pediatric-growth-charts-by-boston-childrens-hospital/id617601789?mt=8

Growth Chart Centers for Disease Control/World Health Organization
https://play.google.com/store/apps/details?id=com.LetsStart.GrowthChart&hl=en

APPENDIX B:

NUTRIENT-RICH FOODS FOR KIDS

(All tables have been adapted from Fearless Feeding: How to Raise Healthy Eaters from High Chair to High School)

Appendix B.1 Calcium-Rich Food Sources for Kids		
Food	**Portion Size**	**Calcium (mg)**
Orange juice, calcium fortified	1 cup	300
Plain yogurt, nonfat	8 ounces	452
Romano cheese	1½ ounces	452
Ricotta cheese, part skim	1/2 cup	337
Yogurt, fruit, low fat	8 ounces	338–384
Mozzarella, part skim	1.5 ounces	333
Sardines, canned in oil, with bones	3 ounces	325
Cheddar cheese	1.5 ounces	307
Low-fat milk (1%)	1 cup	305
Nonfat milk	8 ounces	299
Reduced-fat milk (2%)	8 ounces	293
Low-fat chocolate milk (1%)	1 cup	290
Buttermilk	8 ounces	282–350
Whole milk (3.25%)	8 ounces	276
Reduced fat chocolate milk (2%)	1 cup	272
Tofu, firm, made with calcium sulfate***	1/2 cup	253
Salmon, pink, canned, solids with bone	3 ounces	181
Cottage cheese, 1% milk fat	1 cup	138
Tofu, soft, made with calcium sulfate***	1/2 cup	138
Instant breakfast drink, various flavors and brands, powder prepared with water	8 ounces	105–250
Frozen yogurt, vanilla, soft serve	1/2 cup	103
Ready-to-eat cereal, calcium-fortified	1/2 cup	100–1,000
Turnip greens, fresh, boiled	1/2 cup	99
Kale, fresh, cooked	1/2 cup	94
Kale, raw, chopped	1 cup	90

Appendix B.1 Calcium-Rich Food Sources for Kids (Continued)		
Food	**Portion Size**	**Calcium (mg)**
Ice cream, vanilla	1 cup	84
Soy beverage, calcium-fortified	1/2 cup	80–500
Chinese cabbage, bok choi, raw, shredded	1 cup	74
Bread, white	1 slice	73
Pudding, chocolate, ready to eat, refrigerated	4 ounces	55
Tortilla, corn, ready-to-bake/fry	one 6" diameter	46
Tortilla, flour, ready-to-bake/fry	one 6" diameter	32
Sour cream, reduced fat, cultured	2 tablespoons	31
Bread, whole-wheat	1 slice	30
Broccoli, raw	1/2 cup	21
Cheese, cream, regular	1 tablespoon	14

Appendix B.2 Vitamin D-Rich Food Sources for Kids

Food	Portion Size	Vitamin D (mcg)*
Salmon, sockeye, cooked	3 ounces	19.8
Salmon, smoked	3 ounces	14.5
Salmon, canned	3 ounces	11.6
Rockfish, cooked	3 ounces	6.5
Tuna, light, canned in oil, drained	3 ounces	5.7
Orange juice	1 cup	3.4
Sardine, canned in oil, drained	3 ounces	4.1
Tuna, light, canned in water, drained	3 ounces	3.8
Whole milk	1 cup	3.2
Whole chocolate milk	1 cup	3.2
Reduced fat chocolate milk (2%)	1 cup	3
Milk (nonfat, 1% and 2%)	1 cup	2.9
Low-fat chocolate milk (1%)	1 cup	2.8
Soymilk	1 cup	2.7
Evaporated milk, nonfat	1/2 cup	2.6
Flatfish (flounder and sole), cooked	3 ounces	2.5
Fortified ready-to-eat cereals (various)	3/4–1 1/4 cup (about 1 ounce)	0.9–2.5
Rice drink	1 cup	2.4
Shiitake mushrooms	1/2 cup	0.6
Herring, pickled	3 ounces	2.4
Pork, cooked (various cuts)	3 ounces	0.6–2.2
Cod, cooked	3 ounces	1
Beef liver, cooked	3 ounces	1
Cured ham	3 ounces	0.6–0.8
Egg, hard-boiled	1 large	0.7
Canadian bacon	2 slices (about 1 1/2 ounces)	0.5

1 mcg of vitamin D is equivalent to 40 IU

Appendix B.3 Iron-Rich Food Sources for Kids

Food Sources	Portion Size	Iron (mg)
Heme Iron		
Chicken liver, pan-fried	3 ounces	11
Oysters, canned	3 ounces	5.7
Beef liver, pan-fried	3 ounces	5.2
Beef, chuck, blade roast, lean only, braised	3 ounces	3.1
Turkey, dark meat, roasted	3 ounces	2
Beef, ground, 85% lean, patty, broiled	3 ounces	2.2
Beef, top sirloin, steak, lean only, broiled	3 ounces	1.6
Tuna, light, canned in water	3 ounces	1.3
Turkey, light meat, roasted	3 ounces	1.1
Chicken, dark meat, meat only, roasted	3 ounces	1.1
Chicken, light meat, meat only, roasted	3 ounces	0.9
Tuna, fresh, yellowfin, cooked, dry heat	3 ounces	0.8
Crab, Alaskan king, cooked, moist heat	3 ounces	0.7
Pork, loin chop, broiled	3 ounces	0.7
Shrimp, mixed species, cooked, moist heat	4 large	0.3
Halibut, cooked, dry heat	3 ounces	0.2
Nonheme Iron		
Ready-to-eat cereal, 100% iron fortified	3/4 cup	18
Oatmeal, instant, fortified, prepared with water	1 packet	11
Soybeans, mature, boiled	1 cup	8.8
Lentils, boiled	1 cup	6.6
Beans, kidney, mature, boiled	1 cup	5.2
Beans, lima, large, mature, boiled	1 cup	4.5
Ready-to-eat cereal, 25% iron fortified	3/4 cup	4.5
Black-eyed peas, (cowpeas), mature, boiled	1 cup	4.3
Beans, navy, mature, boiled	1 cup	4.3
Beans, black, mature, boiled	1 cup	3.6
Beans, pinto, mature, boiled	1 cup	3.6
Tofu, raw, firm	1/2 cup	3.4
Spinach, fresh, boiled, drained	1/2 cup	3.2

Appendix B.3 Iron-Rich Food Sources for Kids (Continued)

Food Sources	Portion Size	Iron (mg)
Nonheme Iron		
Spinach, canned, drained solid	1/2 cup	2.5
Spinach, frozen, chopped or leaf, boiled	1/2 cup	1.9
Raisins, seedless, packed	1/2 cup	1.6
Grits, white, enriched, quick, prepared with water	1 cup	1.5
Molasses	1 tablespoon	0.9
Bread, white, commercially prepared	1 slice	0.9
Bread, whole-wheat, commercially prepared	1 slice	0.7

Appendix B.4 Vitamin A-Rich Food Sources for Kids		
Food	**Portion Size**	**vitamin A (IU)**
Selected Animal Sources		
Liver, beef, cooked	3 ounces	22,175
Liver, chicken, cooked	3 ounces	11,329
Milk, nonfat, fortified	1 cup	500
Cheese, cheddar	1 ounce	284
Milk, whole	1 cup	395
Egg, hard-boiled	1 large	260
Selected Plant Sources		
Carrot juice, canned	1/2 cup	22,567
Sweet potato, baked in skin	1 medium	21,909
Carrots, boiled	1/2 cup	13,286
Spinach, frozen, chopped or leaf, boiled	1/2 cup	11,458
Carrots, raw	1/2 cup	9,189
Kale, cooked, boiled	1/2 cup	8,854
Vegetable soup, canned, chunky, ready-to-serve	1 cup	5,878
Cantaloupe, cubes	1 cup	5,411
Lettuce, Romaine, raw	1 cup	4,878
Spinach, raw	1 cup	2,813
Apricots, canned, juice pack	1/2 cup	2,063
Mango, sliced	1 cup	1,785
Peas, frozen, boiled	1/2 cup	1,680
Apricot nectar, canned	1/2 cup	1,652
Oatmeal, instant, fortified, plain, prepared with water	1 cup	1,453
Pepper, sweet, red, raw, sliced	1/2 cup	1,440
Papaya, cubes	1 cup	1,378
Broccoli, boiled	1/2 cup	1,208
Tomato juice, canned	1 cup	1,094
Watermelon, raw	1 cup	865

Appendix B.5 Vitamin-C Rich Food Sources for Kids

Food	Portion Size	Vitamin C (mg)
Red pepper, sweet, raw	1/2 cup	158
Orange juice	3/4 cup	155
Orange	1 medium	117
Grapefruit juice	3/4 cup	117
Kiwifruit	1 medium	107
Green pepper, sweet, raw	1/2 cup	100
Broccoli, cooked	1/2 cup	85
Strawberries, fresh, sliced	1/2 cup	82
Brussels sprouts, cooked	1/2 cup	80
Vegetable juice cocktail	1 cup	67
Grapefruit	1/2 medium	65
Broccoli, raw	1/2 cup	65
Fortified ready-to-eat cereals (various)	3/4 - 1 1/3 cup (~1 ounce)	60-61
Tomato juice	3/4 cup	55
Cantaloupe	1/2 cup	48
Cabbage, cooked	1/2 cup	47
Papaya	1/2 cup	43
Cauliflower, raw	1/2 cup	43
Pineapple	1/2 cup	39
Potato, baked	1 medium	28
Tomato, raw	1 medium	28
Kale, cooked from fresh	1/2 cup	27
Tangerine	1 medium	24
Mango	1/2 cup	23
Spinach, cooked	1/2 cup	15
Green peas, frozen, cooked	1/2 cup	13

Appendix B.6 Zinc-Rich Food Sources for Kids

Food	Portion Size	Zinc (mg)
Oysters, cooked, breaded and fried	3 ounces	493
Beef chuck roast, braised	3 ounces	47
Crab, Alaska king, cooked	3 ounces	43
Beef patty, broiled	3 ounces	35
Breakfast cereal, fortified with 25% of the DV for zinc	3/4 cup	25
Lobster, cooked	3 ounces	23
Pork chop, loin, cooked	3 ounces	19
Baked beans, canned, plain or vegetarian	1/2 cup	19
Chicken, dark meat, cooked	3 ounces	16
Yogurt, fruit, low fat	8 ounces	11
Cashews, dry roasted	1 ounce	11
Chickpeas, cooked	1/2 cup	9
Cheese, Swiss	1 ounce	8
Oatmeal, instant, plain, prepared with water	1 packet	7
Milk, low-fat or non fat	1 cup	7
Almonds, dry roasted	1 ounce	6
Kidney beans, cooked	1/2 cup	6
Chicken breast, roasted, skin removed	1/2 breast	6
Cheese, cheddar or mozzarella	1 ounce	6
Peas, green, frozen, cooked	1/2 cup	3
Flounder or sole, cooked	3 ounces	2

Appendix B.7 DHA-Rich Food Sources for Kids			
Food	**Portion size**	**DHA (mg)**	**ALA (mg)**
Salmon (Atlantic farmed, baked)	3 ounces	1,238	
Salmon (Atlantic wild, baked)	3 ounces	1,215	
Tuna (white, packed in water)	3 ounces	535	
Sardines (packed in oil with bone)	3 ounces	433	
Tuna (light, packed in water)	3 ounces	190	
Tuna (light, packed in oil)	3 ounces	86	
Fortified Eggs	1 egg	50-150	
Fortified milk	8 ounces	32	
Fortified soymilk	8 ounces	32	
Fortified orange juice	8 ounces	20	
Fortified baby foods	3 ounces pureed, 1/4 cup cereal	18	
Fortified Yogurt	4 ounces	16-32	
Walnuts	1/4 cup		627
Flax Cereal	3/4 cup		1,000

Appendix B.8 Vitamin E-Rich Food Sources for Kids

Food	Standard Portion Size	Vitamin E (mg)
Wheat germ oil	1 Tablespoon	20.3
Fortified, ready-to-eat cereals (various)	3⁄4 - 1 1/3 cup (~1 ounce)	3.2-13.5
Sunflower seeds, dry roasted	1 ounce	7.4
Almonds, dry roasted	1 ounce	6.8
Sunflower oil	1 Tablespoon	5.6
Safflower oil	1 Tablespoon	4.6
Hazelnuts, dry roasted	1 ounce	4.3
Mixed nuts, dry roasted	1 ounce	3.1
Peanut butter	2 tablespoons	2.9
Pine nuts	1 ounce	2.7
Canola oil	1 Tbsp	2.4
Peanuts, dry roasted	1 ounce	2.2
Corn oil	1 Tablespoon	1.9
Olive oil	1 Tablespoon	1.9
Spinach, boiled	1/2 cup	1.9
Sardines, canned in oil, drained	3 ounces	1.7
Brazil nuts	1 ounce	1.6
Orange roughy, cooked	3 ounces	1.6
Avocado	1/2 cup	1.5
Broccoli, chopped, boiled	1/2 cup	1.2
Soybean oil	1 Tablespoon	1.1
Kiwifruit	1 medium	1.1
Mango, sliced	1/2 cup	0.7
Tomato, raw	1 medium	0.7
Spinach, raw	1 cup	0.6

APPENDIX C:

PORTION GUIDE FOR KIDS

Portion Guide for Kids					
Foods	**2-3 years**	**4-6 years**	**6-9 years**	**10-12 years**	**13-18 years**
Grains					
Bread, Bagel	¼ -1/2	1 slice, ½	1 slice, ½	1 slice, ½	1 slice, ½
Cold cereal	½ cup	½-1 cup	1 cup	1 cup	1 cup
Cooked cereal Pasta, rice	¼ - ½ cup	½ cup	½ cup	½ cup	½ cup
Crackers	2 - 3	4 - 6	5 – 7	5 – 7	5 - 7
Fruits					
Whole, fresh	½-1 small	½ -1 small	½ -1 cup, 1 medium	1 cup, 1 medium	1 cup, 1 medium
Cooked/canned	1/3 cup	½ cup	½ - 1 cup	1 cup	1 cup
Dried Juice	¼ - 1/3 cup	2 Tbsp. ½ cup	¼ cup ½ cup	¼ cup ½ cup	¼ cup ½ cup
Vegetables					
Whole, fresh Raw, leafy greens	½ small ¼ - ½ cup	½ - 1 small ½ - 1 cup	½ - 1 cup 1 cup	1 cup 1 – 2 cup	1 cup 1 - 2 cup
Cooked/canned	2-3 Tbsp.	¼ -½ cup	½-1 cup	½-1 cup	½-1 cup
Juice	¼ - 1/3 cup	1/3 - ½ cup	½ cup	½ cup	½ cup
Dairy/ Non-Dairy					
Milk or Yogurt	½- ¾ cup	½ - 1 cup	¾ -1 cup	¾ - 1 cup	1 cup
Cheese	½ ounce	¾ ounce	1 - 1 ½ ounce	1 ½ ounce 1/3 c. shred	1 ½ ounce 1/3 c. shred

Foods	2-3 years	4-6 years	6-9 years	10-12 years	13-18 years
Protein					
Beef, poultry, fish	1-2 Tbsp.	1-2 Tbsp.	2 ounce	3 ounce	3 ounce
Beans Nuts, seeds Nut butter	1-2 Tbsp. ¼ oz. 1 – 2 tsp.	2-3 Tbsp. ¼ - ½ oz. 2 – 3 tsp.	¼ cup cooked ½ ounce 1 Tbsp.	¼ cup cooked ½ ounce 1 Tbsp.	¼ cup cooked ½ ounce 1 Tbsp.
Egg	½ - 1	1	1	1	1
Fats					
Butter, margarine	1 tsp.	1 tsp.	1 tsp.	1 tsp.	1 tsp.
Oil	1 tsp.	1 tsp.	1 tsp.	1 tsp.	1 tsp.
Salad dressing Mayonnaise	1-2 tsp.	½ - 1 Tbsp.	1 Tbsp.	1-2 Tbsp.	1-2 Tbsp.

APPENDIX D:

VITAMIN AND MINERAL SUPPLEMENTS

Nature's Plus Animal Parade by Nature's Plus	Chewable MVI + mineral	
Nature's Plus Animal Parade Gold by Nature's Plus	Chewable MVI + mineral	Contains additional EPA and probiotics
Nature's Plus Power Teen (for Him or Her) by Nature's Plus	Chewable MVI + mineral	For teens
Nature's Way Alive Children's Chewable by Nature's Way	Chewable MVI + mineral	
Rainbow Light Kid's One Chewable by Rainbow Light Nutritional Systems	Chewable MVI + mineral	
Flintstones Compete	Chewable MVI + mineral	Can get with iron, too
Dolphin Pals Multivitamin and Minerals by Country Life	Liquid MVI + minerals	
Rainbow Light Gummy Power Sours by Rainbow Light	Gummy MVI + mineral	
Yummi Bears Organics Complete Sugar- Free Multivitamin	Gummy MVI + mineral	
Smarty Pants Gummy Multivitamin with mineral	Gummy MVI + mineral	

APPENDIX E:

COMMERCIAL AND HOMEMADE SUPPLEMENTAL DRINKS

HIGH CALORIE, NUTRIENT DENSE, HOMEMADE SHAKES & SMOOTHIES & COMMERCIALLY-PREPARED OPTIONS

F YOUR CHILD IS UNDERWEIGHT, or unwilling to eat enough at school, try a smoothie or milkshake to bridge the gap in nutrition. Be sure to use high calorie, nutrient-rich ingredients! Try: avocados, full-fat milk and yogurts (if tolerated), bananas, mango, nut butters, whole unsweetened (canned) coconut milk, coconut oil, 100 percent juices and flax seeds, for example.

If allergic to milk, try pea protein based milks (Ripple, eg) or soymilk, as these will best mimic the nutrition of regular milk. Or opt for canned coconut milk or almond milk.

If allergic to peanuts or nuts, substitute SunButter (made from sunflower seeds).

Do not use weight gainer or protein supplement products aimed at adults – they may be too high in protein and may contain questionable, unsafe ingredients for your child.

To sweeten without sugar, try Stevia.

For all milkshake and smoothie recipes, add the liquid ingredients to the blender first, then the solids. You can always add more liquid to achieve the consistency or thickness your child desires.

Vanilla Milkshake
- 1 cup whole milk
- ¼ cup dry milk powder
- ¾ - 1 cup vanilla ice cream

Peanut Butter Banana Yogurt Shake
- 1 cup whole milk
- ½ cup vanilla yogurt
- 1 frozen banana (medium size)
- 2-3 tablespoons peanut butter

Strawberry Frosty

- 1 envelope of Strawberry Instant Breakfast

- 1 cup whole milk

- ¼ cup dry milk powder

- ½ cup strawberry flavored yogurt

- 4-6 ice cubes

Chocolate Peanut Butter Shake

- 1 cup whole milk

- 3 tablespoons cocoa powder or Ovaltine

- 1 heaping tablespoon of peanut butter

- ½ cup vanilla yogurt

- 4-6 ice cubes

Avocado Berry Smoothie

- 1 avocado

- 1 cup frozen raspberries or mixed berries

- 1 cup whole milk

- 1-2 tablespoons honey or maple syrup

Ready-to-Use Commercial Options

- Boost Kid Essentials

- Pediasure

- Ovaltine

- Carnation Instant Breakfast Essentials

- Resource Breeze

- NutriPal Shakes

APPENDIX F:

RESOURCES:TREATMENT, HELPFUL BOOKS, WEBSITES, AND OTHER RESOURCES

Treatment

Find a Dietitian Expert: www.eatright.org/findanexpert/

Find a Feeding Therapist: https://www.feedingmatters.org/families/feeding-services

Find a Psychologist: https://www.psychologytoday.com/us/therapists/

Mealtime Hostage: A closed Facebook group for parents of extreme picky eaters

https://www.facebook.com/mealtimehostage

Books

Helping Your Child with Extreme Picky Eating: A Step-by-Step Guide for Overcoming Selective Eating, Food Aversion, and Feeding Disorders by Katja Rowell, MD & Jenny McGlothlin, MS, CCC-SLP

Conquer Picky Eating for Teens and Adults by Jenny McGlothlin, MS, CCC-SLP and Katja Rowell, MD

From Picky to Powerful: The Mindset, Strategies and Know-How You Need to Empower Your Picky Eater by Maryann Tomovich Jacobsen

Food Chaining by Cheri Fraker, Mark Fishbein, Sybil Cox, and Laura Walbert

Fearless Feeding: How to Raise Healthy Eaters from High Chair to High School, 2nd edition by Jill Castle and Maryann Tomovich Jacobsen

Adventures in Veggieland by Melanie Potock, MA, CCC-SLP

The Calcium Handbook by Jill Castle, MS, RDN

It's Not About the Broccoli by Dina Rose

Child of Mine by Ellyn Satter

Secrets of Feeding a Healthy Family: How to Eat, How to Raise Good Eaters, How to Cook by Ellyn Satter

The Picky Eater Project: 6 Weeks to Happy Family Meals by Natalie Muth and Sally Sampson

Articles and Online Support

Support for Extreme Picky Eating (ARFID):
http://pediatricfeedingnews.com/feeding-therapy-what-to-do-when-you-are-stuck/

ASHA blog: http://www.asha.org/public/speech/swallowing/Feeding-and-Swallowing-Disorders-in-Children/

Mealtime Hostage blog https://mealtimehostage.com/

My Munch Bug blog: https://www.mymunchbug.com/

The Nourished Child Podcast: https://apple.co/2hUj1UA

Real Mom Nutrition with Sally Kuzemchak: https://realmomnutrition.com/

Super Healthy Kids (recipes and meal planning): https://superhealthykids.com/

The Ellyn Satter Institute: https://www.ellynsatterinstitute.org/

Tools:

Try Pods by Brave Plate, LLC: https://www.braveplate.com/

APPENDIX G:

IN THE KITCHEN: TASTE TESTERS

Taste testing is a fun way to give mom or dad feedback about new foods. After you taste this food, put a checkmark in the column that best describes your experience and how you feel about this food.

	Hate	Don't Like	Don't Mind	Like	Love
Appearance (the way it looks)					
Smell					
Flavor/Taste					
Sweetness					
Sour/Bitter/Salty					
Texture (smooth, bumpy, pointy)					
Touch (the way it feels on your hands/mouth)					

APPENDIX H:

MY ONE AND ONLY SLOW COOKER MEAT RECIPE (BEEF, CHICKEN, PORK)

Ingredients:

- 1 large onion (or 2 small)

- 2-3# cut of lean meat (trim any visible fat)

- 3/4 cup of water

- 1 teaspoon Kosher salt

- 1/2 -3/4 teaspoon pepper

Directions:

Cut the onion into quarters and layer on the bottom of the crockpot.

Cut meat (beef, chicken or pork) into 3 or 4 pieces and place atop the onions.

Pour water over the meat and add salt and pepper.

Cover and cook on low for 6-8 hours. Take two forks and shred the meat. Now you're ready to serve!

FUN

EXPLORE

I'M LEARNING TO EAT!

What food is this?

What do you taste?

What do you smell?

Where does this food belong?

How does this food feel?

NO PRESSURE

SMALL AMOUNTS

APPENDIX J:

TRY-IT BITES RECORD

TRY-IT BITES

Where: _____

When: _____

What: Describe below which 3 foods you will try for the week.

Instructions: Try a new food! Tell me how you tried it (lick, kiss, taste, chew, swallow). ↑ means you liked it; ↓ means you didn't like it; →← means you're not sure yet.

Week of:	Food #1:	Food #2:	Food #3:
	Example: macaroni noodle	Spaghetti noodle	Ziti noodle
Monday	↑	→←	↑
Monday			
Tuesday			
Wednesday			
Thursday			
Friday			
Saturday			
Sunday			

TRY NEW FOOD

Week of:	Food #1:	Food #2:	Food #3:
Monday			
Tuesday			
Wednesday			
Thursday			
Friday			
Saturday			
Sunday			

Week of:	Food #1:	Food #2:	Food #3:
Monday			
Tuesday			
Wednesday			
Thursday			
Friday			
Saturday			
Sunday			

TRY NEW FOOD

Week of:	Food #1:	Food #2:	Food #3:
Monday			
Tuesday			
Wednesday			
Thursday			
Friday			
Saturday			
Sunday			

APPENDIX K:

MASTER LIST OF LIKED FOODS

Foods I Tried	Foods I Liked

Foods I Tried	Foods I Liked

NOTES

1. Taylor, C.M., Wernimont, S.M., Northstone, K., et al. (2015) Picky/fussy eating in children: Review of definitions, assessment, prevalence and dietary intakes. *Appetite*, *95*, 349-359.

2. Carruth, B.R., Skinner, J., Houck, K., Moran, J., Coletta, F., Ott, D. (1998) The phenomenon of "picky eater": A behavioral marker in eating patterns of toddlers. *Journal of American College of Nutrition*, *17*, 180-186.

3. Jacobi, C., Agras, W.S., Bryson, S., Hammer, L.D. (2003) Behavioral validation, precursors, and concomitants of picky eating in childhood. *Journal of American Academy of Child and Adolescent Psychiatry*, *42*, 76-84.

4. Dubois, L., Farmer, A.P., Girard, M., Peterson, K. (2007) Preschool children's eating behaviours are related to dietary adequacy and body weight. *European Journal of Clinical Nutrition*, *61*, 846-855.

5. Branen, L., Fletcher, J. (1999). Comparison of college students' current eating habits and recollections of their childhood practices. *Journal of Nutrition Education*, *31*, 304–310.

6. Kennedy, G. A., Wick, M. R., Keel, P. K. (2018) Eating disorders in children: is avoidant-restrictive food intake disorder a feeding disorder or an eating disorder and what are the implications for treatment?. *F1000Research*, *7*, 88. doi:10.12688/f1000research.13110.1

7. Fisher, Martin M. et al. (2014) Characteristics of avoidant/restrictive food intake disorder in children and adolescents: A "new disorder" in DSM-5. *Journal of Adolescent Health*, *55*(1), 49 – 52.

8. De Cosmi, V., Scaglioni, S., Agostoni, C. (2017). Early taste experiences and later food choices. *Nutrients*, *9*(2), 107. doi:10.3390/nu9020107

9. Stein, L. J., Cowart, B. J., Beauchamp, G. K.. (2011) The development of salty taste acceptance is related to dietary experience in human infants: a prospective study. *American Journal of Clinical Nutrition*, *95*(1), 123. DOI: 10.3945/ajcn.111.014282

10. Monell Chemical Senses Center. Children's taste sensitivity and food choices influenced by taste gene. Science Daily. 18 February 2005.

11. Maier-Nöth, A., Schaal, B., Leathwood, P., Issanchou, S. (2016) The lasting influences of early food-related variety experience: A longitudinal study of vegetable acceptance from

5 months to 6 years in two populations. *PLoS ONE*, *11*(3), e0151356. doi.org/10.1371/journal.pone.0151356

12. Goodell, L.S., Johnson, S.L., Antono, A.C. et al. (2017). Strategies low income parents use to overcome their children's food refusal. *Matern Child Health J*, *21*,(68), doi.org/10.1007/s10995-016-2094-x

13. Holley, C. E., Haycraft, E., & Farrow, C. (2015). 'Why don't you try it again?' A comparison of parent led, home based interventions aimed at increasing children's consumption of a disliked vegetable. *Appetite*, *87*, 215-222. doi:10.1016/j.appet.2014.12.216

14. Coulthard, H., Harris, G., & Fogel, A. (2014). Exposure to vegetable variety in infants weaned at different ages. *Appetite*, *78*, 89-94. doi:10.1016/j.appet.2014.03.021.

15. Mallan, K. M. et al. (2016) The relationship between number of fruits, vegetables, and noncore foods tried at age 14 months and food preferences, dietary intake patterns, fussy eating behavior, and weight status at age 3.7 years. *Journal of the Academy of Nutrition and Dietetics*, *116*(4), 630 – 637.

16. Coulthard, H., Harris, G., & Emmett, P. (2009). Delayed introduction of lumpy foods to children during the complementary feeding period affects child's food acceptance and feeding at 7 years of age. *Maternal & Child Nutrition*, *5*, 75–85.

17. Finn, K., Callen, C., Bhatia, J., Reidy, K., Bechard, L. J., & Carvalho, R. (2017). Importance of dietary sources of iron in infants and toddlers: Lessons from the FITS study. *Nutrients*, *9*(7), 733. doi:10.3390/nu9070733

18. Wagner, C. L., Greer, F. R., & Section on Breastfeeding and Committee on Nutrition. (2008). Clinical report: Prevention of rickets and vitamin D deficiency in infants, children, and adolescents. *Pediatrics*, *122*, 1142–1152.

19. Ceglie G, Macchiarulo G, Marchili MR, et al. (2018) Scurvy: still a threat in the well-fed first world? *Archives of Disease in Childhood*, Published Online First. doi: 10.1136/archdischild-2018-315496

20. Fisher, J. O., & Kral, T.V.E. (2008). Super-size me: Portion size effects on young children's eating. *Physiology & Behavior*, *94*, 39–47.

21. Satter, E. (1990). The feeding relationship: Problems and interventions. *J Pediatrics*, *117*, S181–S189.

22. van der Horst, K. & Sleddens, E.F.C. (2017). Parenting styles, feeding styles and food-related parenting practices in relation to toddlers' eating styles: A cluster-analytic approach. *PLoS ONE*, *12*(5), e0178149. doi.org/10.1371/journal.pone.0178149

23. Butte, N. F. (2009). Impact of infant feeding practices on childhood obesity. *The Journal of Nutrition, 139*, 412S–416S.

24. Slaughter, C. W., & Bryant, A. H. (2004). Hungry for love: The feeding relationship in the psychological development of young children. *The Permanente Journal, 8*(1), 23–29.

25. Wood, A. C., Momin, S., Senn, M., & Hughes, S. O. (2018). Pediatric Eating Behaviors as the Intersection of Biology and Parenting: Lessons from the Birds and the Bees. *Current Nutrition Reports, 7*(1), 1-9. doi:10.1007/s13668-018-0223-4 12

26. Orrell-Valente, J. K., Hill, L. G., Brechwald, W. A., Dodge, K. A., Pettit G. S., & Bates, J. E. (2007). "Just three more bites": An observational analysis of parents' socialization of children's eating at mealtime. *Appetite, 48*, 37–45.

27. Vaughn, A. E., Ward, D. S., Fisher, J. O., Faith, M. S., Hughes, S. O., Kremers, S. P., Power, T. G., et al. (2016). Fundamental constructs in food parenting practices: A content map to guide future research. *Nutrition Reviews, 74*(2), 98-117. doi:10.1093/nutrit/nuv061

28. Scaglioni, S., De Cosmi, V., Ciappolino, V., Parazzini, F., Brambilla, P., & Agostoni, C. (2018). Factors Influencing Children's Eating Behaviours. *Nutrients, 10*(6), 706. http://doi.org/10.3390/nu10060706

29. Blissett, J., Fogel, A. (2013). Intrinsic and extrinsic influences on children's acceptance of new foods. *Physiology & Behavior. 121*(10), 89-95. doi.org/10.1016/j.physbeh.2013.02.013

30. Warren, J. M., Smith, N., & Ashwell, M. (2017). A structured literature review on the role of mindfulness, mindful eating and intuitive eating in changing eating behaviours: Effectiveness and associated potential mechanisms. *Nutrition Research Reviews, 30*(2), 272-283. doi:10.1017/s0954422417000154

31. Chu, Y.L., Farmer, A., Fung, C., Kuhle, S., Storey, K.E., Veugelers, P.J. (2012) Involvement in home meal preparation is associated with food preference and self-efficacy among Canadian children. *Public Health Nutrition*, DOI: 10.1017/S1368980012001218

32. Lumeng, J.C., Miller, A.L., Appugliese, D., Rosenblum, K., Kaciroti, N. (2018). Picky eating, pressuring feeding, and growth in toddlers. *Appetite. 123*, 299-305. https://doi.org/10.1016/j.appet.2017.12.020

33. Batsell, W.R., Brown, A.S., Ansfield, M.E., Paschall, G.Y. (2002). "You will eat all of that!": A retrospective analysis of forced consumption episodes. *Appetite. 38*(3), 211-219. doi.org/10.1006/appe.2001.0482

ABOUT THE AUTHOR

Jill Castle is one of the nation's premier childhood nutrition experts. Known as a paradigm shifter who blends current research, practical application, and common sense, Jill inspires audiences to think differently about feeding children. From babies to teens, Jill takes a unique, "whole-child" approach to showcase food, feeding, and childhood development as the secret ingredients to raising a healthy child.

A sought-after speaker, advisor, and media contributor, Jill has inspired TEDx, American Academy of Pediatrics, WIC, university groups, and a range of nutrition, medical, government, and parent audiences. Jill is on the Board of Advisors of Parents Magazine, and is scientific advisor to a handful of privately held child nutrition companies.

She is the author of *Eat Like a Champion*, *The Smart Mom's Guide to Starting Solids*, *Try New Food*, and co-author of *Fearless Feeding*. She pens *The Nourished Child* blog, interviews experts on her podcast of the same name, and regularly contributes to US News & World Report's *For Parents* blog. She has appeared in The New York Times, WebMD, Fast Company, USA Today, CNN, the Wall Street Journal, Fox and Friends, NBC-CT, and Parents Magazine.

Jill Castle has practiced as a registered dietitian/nutritionist in the field of pediatric nutrition for over 27 years. Formerly a clinical pediatric dietitian at Massachusetts General Hospital and Boston Children's Hospital, Jill currently works as a private practitioner, online educator, consultant, and speaker.

Jill lives in Connecticut with her husband, four children, and two dogs. To learn more about Jill, read her blog, listen to her podcast, or to work with her, go to www.JillCastle.com.

IDEAS, INSIGHTS, AND INSPIRATION

_____

_____

_____

_____

_____

_____

_____

_____

_____

_____

_____

_____

_____

_____

_____

_____

_____

_____

_____

_____

_____

_____

_____

Made in the USA
San Bernardino, CA
24 February 2020

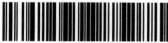